EVALUATING CAPACITY TO WAIVE MIRANDA RIGHTS

BEST PRACTICES IN FORENSIC MENTAL HEALTH ASSESSMENT

Series Editors

Thomas Grisso, Alan M. Goldstein, and Kirk Heilbrun

Series Advisory Board

Paul Appelbaum, Richard Bonnie, and John Monahan

Titles in the Series

Foundations of Forensic Mental Health Assessment, *Kirk Heilbrun, Thomas Grisso, and Alan M. Goldstein*

Criminal Titles

Evaluation of Competence to Stand Trial, *Patricia A. Zapf and Ronald Roesch*

Evaluation of Criminal Responsibility, *Ira K. Packer*

Evaluating Capacity to Waive Miranda Rights, *Alan M. Goldstein and Naomi E. Sevin Goldstein*

Evaluation of Sexually Violent Predators, *Philip H. Witt and Mary Alice Conroy*

Evaluation for Risk of Violence in Adults, *Kirk Heilbrun*

Jury Selection, *Margaret Bull Kovera and Brian L. Cutler*

Evaluation for Capital Sentencing, *Mark D. Cunningham*

Eyewitness Identification, *Brian L. Cutler and Margaret Bull Kovera*

Civil Titles

Evaluation of Capacity to Consent to Treatment and Research, *Scott Y. H. Kim*

Evaluation for Guardianship, *Eric Y. Drogin and Curtis L. Barrett*

Evaluation for Personal Injury Claims, *Andrew W. Kane and Joel Dvoskin*

Evaluation for Civil Commitment, *Debra Pinals and Douglas Mossman*

Evaluation for Harassment and Discrimination Claims, *William Foote and Jane Goodman-Delahunty*

Evaluation of Workplace Disability, *Lisa D. Piechowski*

Juvenile and Family Titles

Evaluation for Child Custody, *Geri S.W. Fuhrmann*

Evaluation of Juveniles' Competence to Stand Trial, *Ivan Kruh and Thomas Grisso*

Evaluation for Risk of Violence in Juveniles, *Robert Hoge and D. A. Andrews*

Evaluation for Child Protection, *Karen S. Budd, Jennifer Clark, Mary Connell, and Kathryn Kuehnle*

Evaluation for Disposition and Transfer of Juvenile Offenders, *Randall T. Salekin*

EVALUATING CAPACITY TO WAIVE MIRANDA RIGHTS

ALAN M. GOLDSTEIN

NAOMI E. SEVIN GOLDSTEIN

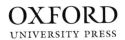

OXFORD
UNIVERSITY PRESS

2010

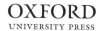

OXFORD
UNIVERSITY PRESS

Oxford University Press

Oxford University Press, Inc., publishes works that further
Oxford University's objective of excellence
in research, scholarship, and education.

Oxford New York
Auckland   Cape Town   Dar es Salaam   Hong Kong   Karachi
Kuala Lumpur   Madrid   Melbourne   Mexico City   Nairobi
New Delhi   Shanghai   Taipei   Toronto

With offices in
Argentina   Austria   Brazil   Chile   Czech Republic   France   Greece
Guatemala   Hungary   Italy   Japan Poland   Portugal   Singapore
South Korea   Switzerland   Thailand   Turkey   Ukraine   Vietnam

Library of Congress Cataloging-in-Publication Data

Goldstein, Alan M.
Evaluating capacity to waive Miranda rights / Alan M. Goldstein &
Naomi E. Sevin Goldstein.
p. cm.—(Best practices in forensic mental health assessment)
Includes bibliographical references and index.
ISBN 978-0-19-536617-4
1. Right to counsel—United States. 2. Self-incrimination—United States.
3. Capacity and disability—United S   KF   sychiatry—United
States. 5. Police questioning—Unite   9625   in, Naomi E. Sevin.
II. Title.   .G65
KF9625.G65 2010   2010
345.73'056—dc22

                                              2010003763

9 8 7 6 5 4 3 2 1

Printed in the United States of Americ
on acid-free paper

About Best Practices in Forensic Mental Health Assessment

The recent growth of the fields of forensic psychology and forensic psychiatry has created a need for this book series describing best practices in forensic mental health assessment (FMHA). Currently, forensic evaluations are conducted by mental health professionals for a variety of criminal, civil, and juvenile legal questions. The research foundation supporting these assessments has become broader and deeper in recent decades. Consensus has become clearer on the recognition of essential requirements for ethical and professional conduct. In the larger context of the current emphasis on "empirically supported" assessment and intervention in psychiatry and psychology, the specialization of FMHA has advanced sufficiently to justify a series devoted to best practices. Although this series focuses mainly on evaluations conducted by psychologists and psychiatrists, the fundamentals and principles offered also apply to evaluations conducted by clinical social workers, psychiatric nurses, and other mental health professionals.

This series describes "best practice" as empirically supported (when the relevant research is available), legally relevant, and consistent with applicable ethical and professional standards. Authors of the books in this series identify the approaches that seem best, while incorporating what is practical and acknowledging that best practice represents a goal to which the forensic clinician should aspire, rather than a standard that can always be met. The American Academy of Forensic Psychology assisted the editors in enlisting the consultation of board-certified forensic psychologists specialized in each topic area. Board-certified forensic psychiatrists were also consultants on many of the volumes. Their comments on the manuscripts helped to ensure that the methods described in these volumes represent a generally accepted view of best practice.

The series' authors were selected for their specific expertise in a particular area. At the broadest level, however, certain general principles apply to all types of forensic evaluations. Rather than repeat those fundamental principles in every volume, the series offers them in the first volume, *Foundations of Forensic Mental Health Assessment*. Reading the first book, followed by a specific topical book, will provide the reader both the general principles that the specific topic shares with all forensic evaluations and those that are particular to the specific assessment question.

The specific topics of the 19 books were selected by the series editors as the most important and oft-considered areas of forensic assessment conducted by mental health professionals and behavioral scientists. Each of the 19 topical books is organized according to a common template. The authors address the applicable legal context, forensic mental health concepts, and empirical foundations and limits in the "Foundation" part of the book. They then describe preparation for the evaluation, data collection, data interpretation, and report writing and testimony in the "Application" part of the book. This creates a fairly uniform approach to considering these areas across different topics. All authors in this series have attempted to be as concise as possible in addressing best practice in their area. In addition, topical volumes feature elements to make them user friendly in actual practice. These elements include boxes that highlight especially important information, relevant case law, best-practice guidelines, and cautions against common pitfalls. A glossary of key terms is also provided in each volume.

We hope the series will be useful for different groups of individuals. Practicing forensic clinicians will find succinct, current information relevant to their practice. Those who are in training to specialize in forensic mental health assessment (whether in formal training or in the process of respecialization) should find helpful the combination of broadly applicable considerations presented in the first volume together with the more specific aspects of other volumes in the series. Those who teach and supervise trainees can offer these volumes as a guide for practices to which the trainee can aspire. Researchers and scholars interested in FMHA best practice may find researchable ideas, particularly on topics that have received insufficient research attention to date. Judges and attorneys with questions about FMHA best practice will find these books relevant and concise. Clinical and forensic administrators who run agencies, court clinics, and hospitals in which litigants are assessed may also use some of the books in this series to establish expectancies for evaluations performed by professionals in their agencies.

We also anticipate that the 19 specific books in this series will serve as reference works that help courts and attorneys evaluate the quality of forensic mental health professionals' evaluations. A word of caution is in order, however. These volumes focus on best practice, not what is minimally acceptable legally or ethically. Courts involved in malpractice litigation, or ethics committees or licensure boards considering complaints, should not expect that materials describing best practice easily or necessarily translate into the minimally acceptable professional conduct that is typically at issue in such proceedings.

This book focuses on information critical to those forensic mental health professionals who are asked to evaluate the capacity of a juvenile or an adult defendant to make a valid waiver of *Miranda* rights. The criteria for a valid waiver—knowingly, intelligently, and voluntarily—are defined. Landmark legal cases related to this area of forensic mental health practice are reviewed. Specific ethical issues that may arise when conducting these assessments are discussed, along with suggestions to address and resolve them. Research on those factors such as age, sex, level of intelligence, prior experience with the legal system, the presence of mental illness, and traits such as suggestibility is reviewed in light of their potential impact on a defendant's likelihood of waiving his or her Constitutional rights. Methodology that experts should consider when evaluating such cases is reviewed, including the role of forensic assessment instruments, and ways of addressing the possibility that the defendant is exaggerating or malingering limitations in comprehending these rights. How the expert interprets numerous sources of data to form an opinion and present the findings in a focused, coherent report and in testimony is considered.

Kirk Heilbrun
Thomas Grisso
Alan M. Goldstein

Acknowledgments

The right to remain silent and the right to consult an attorney when arrested is more than just a legal technicality. These are fundamental rights that are cornerstones of our system of justice; they reflect our country's most sacred values: a sense of fairness and a search for justice. We express our admiration and gratitude to those law enforcement officers, attorneys, and judges who take these principles seriously.

We want to thank Tom Grisso for his pioneering work in the field of forensic mental health assessment and for his contributions in making the evaluation of the capacity to waive *Miranda* rights an objective, data-based area of practice. Kirk Heilbrun and Tom Grisso served as editors for this volume. Their suggestions were always on target and were of tremendous value as we revised this manuscript. Greg DeClue was the external reviewer of our manuscript and we thank him for his willingness to take on that task. Our gratitude to Cristina Wojdylo, our developmental editor at Oxford University Press, for her contribution in making this a user-friendly, readable book. We are appreciative for the support and gentle guidance of Regan Hofmann, Editor at Oxford University Press.

We want to dedicate this book to our families. Alan Goldstein is grateful and in awe of his coauthor and daughter, Naomi, who always takes his long, complex sentences and translates them into a language others can understand. To my wife Paula and my other daughter, Marion, thank you for trying to keep me sane. To my sons-in-law, Josh Sevin and Jon Feldman, I cannot begin to express my gratitude for your sense of ethics and values (and your choices of wives). To Maia and Hillary, my amazing granddaughters, I love you and hope that the rights we enjoy today remain as deeply rooted and protected when you have grandchildren.

Naomi Goldstein is deeply grateful to her father and coauthor, Alan Goldstein, for modeling the perfect balance between work and family, and for his incredible patience in awaiting drafts of chapters—there are not many daughters who would want to coauthor a book with their fathers, and this was a real treat. To my husband, Josh, who challenges my thinking, encourages my pursuits, and offers endless love and support. To my daughters, Hillary and Maia, who bring me such joy—may you never need first-hand knowledge of your *Miranda* rights! To my mother, Paula, who provides unwavering encouragement, and to my sister, Marion, and brother-in-law, Jon, who offer humor at the most needed times. To my many mentors over the years who have provided me with outstanding research training and contributed to my thinking about *Miranda*-related issues, most notably David Arnold, Tom Grisso, Kirk Heilbrun, and Lois Oberlander Condie. And, importantly, to my many graduate and undergraduate students over the past decade that have played key roles in my *Miranda* rights research, especially Rachel Kalbeitzer, Christina Riggs Romaine, Marty Strachan, and Heather Zelle—I thank you for your work, ideas, and collaboration.

Contents

FOUNDATION

The Legal Context | 1

Criminal defendants' rights to avoid self-incrimination and be represented by counsel are core foundations of the U.S. legal system. These rights, provided under the Constitution's Fifth and Sixth Amendments, are often referred to as *Miranda* rights, after the widely recognized Supreme Court case (*Miranda v. Arizona*, 1966) in which their constitutionality was upheld. In this chapter, we consider (1) the sociolegal purpose and history of *Miranda* rights; (2) the distinction between evaluations that inform courts' decisions about the validity of *Miranda* waivers and evaluations of the validity of confessions; and (3) the distinctions between evaluating capacities to have waived *Miranda* rights in juvenile and adult court cases. We review the legal standards used by judges when determining the validity of waivers, as these standards guide our forensic mental health assessments. Landmark decisions, both pre- and post-*Miranda*, are discussed. We describe the legal procedures for cases in which questions have been raised about the validity of defendants' *Miranda* waivers, including such procedures as raising the psycho-legal issue, the admissibility of testimony, and the legal consequences of judges' decisions on the suppression of confessions.

In subsequent chapters, we present several additional considerations. We discuss mental health concepts relevant to conducting assessments of defendants' capacities to have waived *Miranda* rights, including the psychological operationalization of the legal criteria required to execute valid waivers. We describe the research on juveniles' and adults' capacities to waive rights and on the forensic assessment instruments used to objectively evaluate understanding and appreciation of such rights. We discuss how to prepare for an examination of capacity to have waived rights; this section includes a description of data that should be collected during examinations, consistent with best practices, and guidance on how to analyze and interpret the multiple sources of information that must be considered when forming an opinion on this psycholegal issue. Finally, we describe the product of the evaluative process—the written report and testimony.

Although this book comprises seven separate chapters, each must be read within the context of the others. The forensic mental health practitioner must understand the information in all of the chapters in order to responsibly use the material provided in any one chapter. For instance, when the forensic mental health practitioner is accepting the initial referral, she is already obtaining information relevant to testimony. Similarly, when selecting reliable, valid methodology in preparation for the evaluation, the forensic mental health expert must already understand the legal constructs and their corresponding psychological concepts. Furthermore, to meaningfully interpret the assessment data, the expert must be aware of the extant research on juvenile and adult capacities to comprehend their rights and execute valid waivers. These data and the evaluator's hypotheses may develop into opinions that will be presented in the report and, possibly, at a suppression hearing. Thus, although there is a "flow" from chapter to chapter and a distinction in the focus between chapters, we integrated the content across chapters for consistency with practice standards that require knowledge and integration of information across stages of the evaluation process.

In this book, we use "he" and "she" in alternate chapters in order to avoid the bulky "he/she" or "(s)he." Examples cited throughout this book may be based on actual cases. When they are, the names of defendants and other parties have been altered, as have facts and locations that could reveal the identities of people involved. Such examples are important because this book, like others in the Oxford series "Best Practices in Forensic Mental Health Assessment," seeks to illustrate applied material in a concise and practical way. Consider the following case example, in which all names and identifying information have been changed.

Mark Woods, age 14, was arrested and charged with sexually abusing a neighbor's 8-year-old daughter. After receiving authorization from Mark's mother to speak with her son, a detective questioned Mark at school. In the Guidance Office, with his guidance counselor present, Mark was read his *Miranda* rights, told the detective he understood them, and initialed a one-page form listing his rights. He then began to answer the detective's questions. Although he first denied involvement in the crime, after one hour Mark gave an oral statement admitting he had accidentally touched the victim's undergarments. He was arrested, charged with Sexual Abuse, and, the next morning, released to his parents' custody. Two days later, when re-interviewed by the same detective, Mark admitted that he had purposefully put his hand inside the victim's panties and rubbed her vagina. His parents were told of their son's confession and decided that Mark should be represented by an attorney.

Mr. Michaels, the assigned defense counsel, spoke with Mark and later with his parents. The Woods parents told Mr. Michaels that when Mark was four, he could not sit still, had trouble paying attention, and was diagnosed with attention deficit hyperactivity disorder by his pediatrician. Despite Mark's receiving medication for this condition, the Woods parents recalled, his concentration difficulties continued and quickly affected his academic performance.

The lawyer learned that, in the first grade, his client was classified as Learning Disabled and placed in Special Education. Mark was held back in both the second and fifth grades and continued in special education classes until the time of his arrest; in those last two years, he participated in a vocationally oriented program. His scores on standardized tests of reading comprehension, spelling, and math fell far below grade level, with Mark falling progressively further behind as he advanced in school. When speaking with his client, the attorney noted Mark's difficulty paying attention and the frequency with which Mark answered questions in an irrelevant fashion. When asked to describe the interrogation itself, Mark's answers were vague, simplistic, and concrete. Of most significance to his attorney,

Mark did not appear capable of explaining the meaning of the rights he had been read and had waived.

Despite Mark's voluntary statement, videotaped confession, and acknowledgment that he had understood each of his rights, his attorney questioned whether his client had actually grasped the meaning of the Constitutional protections he so quickly waived. Recognizing the significance that Mark's confession would have at trial (Mark was to be tried as an adult in this jurisdiction because of the nature of the offense), his lawyer sought to have the judge exclude his client's *inculpatory statements* from trial.

The Fifth Amendment of the U.S. Constitution protects the right of those arrested to remain silent—to refuse to speak to interrogators without presumption of guilt. The Sixth Amendment constitutionally guarantees the right to be represented by a lawyer, not only at trial, but before and during interrogation as well. Mark's lawyer believed that, at the time his client waived these rights, he was unable to comprehend their meaning and, therefore, was unable invoke these rights and benefit from their protections. Mark was referred for forensic mental health assessment of those factors that may have affected his capacity to have waived his rights in a legally valid manner.

This volume will consider relevant case law, research, and specialized methodology that forensic mental health evaluators need to be familiar with in order to conduct assessments similar to that which is required in Mark's case. The redacted assessment report on this case can be found on the series companion Web site at www.oup.com/us/forensicassessment. It is intended to demonstrate how the material presented in this book contributes to a focused, relevant report on a range of issues related to the capacity of a defendant to have provided a knowing, intelligent, and voluntary waiver of his rights.

Sociolegal Purpose and History

Police are invested in protecting the public and maintaining law and order. Part of that charge involves conducting investigations when crimes have been committed, identifying and questioning potential suspects, and making arrests. As part of this process, in order to increase the likelihood of convictions, police attempt to obtain confessions from suspects.

Significance of Confessions in the Legal Process

Prosecutors consider a suspect's confession to be a critical component of a case. "A defendant's confession often serves as the most persuasive evidence in criminal trials, and is particularly influential when it serves as the sole or primary source of evidence offered by the prosecution" (Oberlander, Goldstein, & Goldstein, 2003, p. 335). A confession, if offered as evidence at trial, is likely to have a profound effect on the outcome of the case. As such, some defense attorneys may challenge incriminating statements made by their clients with one of two arguments: (1) the confession was false (i.e., inaccurate information was physically or emotionally coerced, it was a fantasy on the part of defendant, inaccurate information was provided as a result of the client's suggestibility) or (2) even if the defendant's confession were true, it was illegally obtained and should be excluded at trial.

THE IMPORTANCE OF *MIRANDA* RIGHTS

In 1884, the U.S. Supreme Court commented on the significance of a confession: "A confession, if freely and voluntarily made, is evidence of the most satisfactory character. Such a confession is deserving of the highest credit, because it is presumed to flow from the strongest sense of guilt, and therefore it is admitted as proof of the crime . . . " (*Hopt v. Territory of Utah*, 1884). In this and other pre-*Miranda* cases, a primary focus of the Court was on issues related to the voluntariness of the confession, suggesting that coerced confessions should raise questions about truthfulness (DeClue, 2005).

In *Miranda v. Arizona*, the Court sought to protect suspects' vulnerability by requiring police to inform those under arrest or in police custody of the right to remain silent and right to have an attorney present, not only at trial, but during an interrogation as well. For a suspect to provide a legally valid waiver of rights it is not sufficient for police to have merely read these warnings—the suspect also must be able to knowingly, intelligently, and

CASE LAW

Miranda v.
Arizona (1966)

● The U.S. Supreme Court held that police must inform individuals under arrest or in police custody of their rights to remain silent and to have an attorney present before and during questioning.

voluntarily waive them. In other words, the suspect must understand the basic meaning of the rights to silence and counsel, appreciate their significance and the consequences of waiving them, and waive the rights free from police coercion.

Over the years, courts have identified a number of factors that may raise questions about the legality of a confession, based on *Miranda* and other cases described in this book. If, at a pretrial suppression hearing, testimony is offered about the presence and effects of one or more of these factors on the providing of a *Miranda* rights waiver, a judge may rule that the incriminating statements were obtained in violation of the law. Such a ruling results in the exclusion of the confession as evidence at trial; if the rights to silence and counsel were not validly waived, the confession is considered "fruit of the poisonous tree," legally contaminated by the process by which it was obtained. Many of the factors (e.g., intellectual impairment, neurological dysfunction, developmental immaturity) that can affect whether the waiver was made in a knowing, intelligent, and voluntary manner (see chapter 3 for a review of these factors) can be assessed by forensic mental health professionals. As a result, forensic psychologists and psychiatrists may be asked by attorneys to evaluate their clients' capacities to have waived their *Miranda* rights—could the client have made a knowing, intelligent, and voluntary rights waiver at the time she provided the incriminating information; if not, what factors interfered with the capacity to provide that valid rights wavier?

The authors of this volume remind the reader that the trial judge determines if the rights were waived in a legally valid fashion. As forensic mental health professionals, we evaluate *capacities* that are relevant to or can impact the defendant's abilities to provide a valid waiver of rights. Throughout this book, we use the term "validity of waivers" or "valid waiver" as legal concepts, constructs that include the knowing, intelligent, and voluntary requirements for a legally valid waiver; validity, in this context, does not refer to the psychometric concept of validity nor does it suggest an ultimate opinion on the part of the expert.

Not all suspects are required to receive their *Miranda* warnings prior to providing a confession. For example, confessions that are spontaneously given (the individual voluntarily walks into a police station and confesses to a crime she has committed) are not suppressed under *Miranda* because a reading of rights is not required. Similarly, if a person, who is not considered to be a suspect in the case, spontaneously confesses while being interviewed by police, the court will probably not suppress the confession. Melton, Petrila, Poythress, and Slobogin (2007) reviewed a number of other, noncustodial situations in which courts ruled that *Miranda* warnings need not be given prior to interrogation. However, when questioned while in police custody (or in a situation that a reasonable person would consider police custody), warnings are required (Grisso, 1998). Factors considered by courts in determining whether one should have known they were in police custody include "time elapsed between arrest and confession, whether the confession was made between arrest and arraignment, and whether the defendant knew he or she was a suspect" (Oberlander, Goldstein, & Goldstein, 2003, p. 338). Warnings also must be administered when the police intend to use a confession that they may obtain as evidence at trial (Oberlander, 1998; Oberlander & Goldstein, 2001).

THE ISSUE OF FAIRNESS

In *Miranda v. Arizona*, the U.S. Supreme Court reviewed *Criminal Interrogations and Confessions* (Inbau & Reid, 1962), a text commonly used to train police interrogators to question suspects and obtain confessions. The introduction to this text cautions interrogators to be careful not to increase the likelihood of obtaining false confessions. However, most of the text focuses on methods of eliciting confessions, including techniques designed to take advantage of suspects' weaknesses, discourage suspects' questions about whether they should retain legal counsel, minimize the perceived seriousness of the crime, maximize perceptions of penalties if suspects do not cooperate with interrogators, use non-excessive restraint and food and sleep deprivation, and, in general, wear down the suspects' wills so that they will cooperate with police, answer questions, and provide confessions.

The *Miranda* Court concluded that, in the interests of fairness, there was a need to "level the playing field" between police and suspects. That is, frightened suspects, isolated from family, who are subjected to these interrogation methods might very well disregard their constitutionally guaranteed rights to silence and legal representation. The Court opined that a balance must be struck between the needs of police to question suspects and the protection of suspects' rights. In *Dickerson v. United States* (2000), a landmark case reaffirming the *Miranda* requirement of administering warnings, the Court reiterated its concern about the inherently coercive nature of custodial interrogations and the potential blurring of boundaries between voluntary and involuntary statements.

Historical Background of the Right to Silence

During the Spanish Inquisition, confessions were sometimes obtained through threats of physical torture and death. In *Brown v. Walker* (1896), the U.S. Supreme Court noted that "manifestly unjust methods of interrogating accused persons" were common throughout the European continent. In sixteenth-century England, upon arrest, suspects would be brought before a judge and questioned by that judge. Either the incriminating statements were presented at trial or the defendant's failure to answer the judge's questions was admitted as evidence. The *Brown* decision noted that, historically, the "inquisitorial character [of the system] to press unduly the witness, to browbeat him if he be timid or reluctant, to push him into a corner, and to entrap him into fatal contradictions, which is so painfully evident in many of the earlier state trials . . . made the system so odious as to give rise to a demand for its total abolition." Initially, changes in interrogation procedures were based not upon statues or judicial opinion, but rather "upon a general and silent acquiescence of the courts in a popular demand [sic]" (*Brown v. Walker*, 1896).

By the nineteenth century, the Summary Jurisdiction Act of 1848 prohibited judges in England from questioning detainees about crimes they may have committed. The investigative process was removed from the function of the judiciary. Judges' Rules developed, suggesting that police officers should warn suspects that they had the right not to answer questions about a crime. These procedural rules were later adopted as required police procedures (Law Reform Commission of South Wales, 1998; Wood & Crawford, 1989).

British common law on the right to silence was incorporated into the Fifth Amendment of the U.S. Constitution. "So deeply did the inequities of the ancient system impress themselves upon the minds of the American colonists that the States, with one accord, made a denial of the right to question an accused person a part of their fundamental law, so that a maxim, which in England was a mere rule of evidence, became clothed in this country with the impregnability of a constitutional enactment" (*Brown v. Walker*, 1896). The right to remain silent during police interrogation evolved to also encompass the right not to offer testimony against oneself at trial. If a detective was expected to warn suspects that anything a suspect said could be used against her in court, it followed that defendants should not be compelled to testify in court about their involvement in the alleged offense (Melton et al., 2007; Otto & Goldstein, 2005). These rights, initially established by the Constitution, were further elaborated upon by the Court in *Miranda v. Arizona*. In Canada, suspects and defendants are similarly protected under the Charter Rights.

False Confessions

The Court has established a clear distinction between legal questions related to the validity of *Miranda* waivers and the consideration of circumstances that might have helped elicit a false confession. In *Crane v. Kentucky* (1986), the U.S. Supreme Court considered the case of a petitioner, who at age 16, was charged with the murder of a liquor store clerk during the course of a robbery. Defense counsel moved to have her client's confession suppressed, claiming that it was not voluntarily obtained. At a pretrial hearing, the judge ruled that the statement had been voluntarily given and denied the motion to suppress. At trial, Crane's lawyer attempted to introduce evidence for the jury to consider that would argue that the interrogative circumstances surrounding the confession were such that the client's incriminating statement should not be believed. The judge did not allow such testimony, reasoning that the decision had already been rendered at the preliminary hearing—that the confession was voluntarily obtained. Crane was found guilty and sentenced to 40 years in prison. The Supreme Court of Kentucky considered the appeal and affirmed the trial judge's decision to exclude such testimony at trial.

However, in a unanimous decision, the U.S. Supreme Court reversed the Kentucky appeal court's decision. In *Crane v. Kentucky*, writing for the Court, Justice O'Connor ruled that a defendant has the right to offer evidence that may raise questions about the credibility of a confession, reasoning that the circumstances under which the statement was obtained (i.e., physical and psychological environment of the interrogation) are relevant to the statement's credibility; as such, defendants must be allowed to challenge the trustworthiness of the confessions they provided. Relevant factors cited in this specific case included the size of the interrogation room, the lack of windows, the protracted period of questioning, a claim that as many as six police officers had surrounded Crane during the interrogation, the denial of Crane's request to call his mother, and a claim that Crane had been "badgered" into providing a false confession.

In a strongly worded decision, the Court found that "evidence bearing on the voluntariness of a confession and evidence bearing on its credibility fall in conceptually distinct and mutually exclusive categories." Justice O'Connor wrote, "Especially since neither the Supreme Court of Kentucky in its opinion, nor the respondent in its argument to the Court, has advanced any rational justification for the wholesale exclusion of this body of potentially exculpatory evidence, the decision . . . must be reversed." As such, trial courts must allow testimony, including opinions from forensic mental health experts, that address the issue of false confessions—even if

CASE LAW

*Crane v.
Kentucky* (1986)

● The U.S. Supreme
Court ruled that
defendants must be
allowed to challenge
the trustworthiness of
the confessions they
provided.

the court held, at a pretial hearing, that the confession was voluntary obtained and admissible.

DeClue (2005) identified three distinct forensic contexts in which a mental health professional might conduct an evaluation of "voluntariness." When assessing voluntariness, he reported that, first, a forensic mental health professional might assess the validity of a *Miranda* waiver and provide information to help a judge determine whether the defendant waived his *rights* voluntarily. Second, DeClue indicated that, consistent with *Crane v. Kentucky* (described previously), forensic experts can be asked to evaluate factors that may have contributed to a defendant offering a *coerced confession*. He also described a third issue related to voluntariness—a forensic evaluator might evaluate the veracity of a confession, that is, whether the statement provided by the defendant was true or false.

This book clearly emphasized the first context cited by DeClue. It describes the standards of practice in assessing defendants' capacities to have provided a valid waiver of *Miranda* rights. It does not focus on voluntariness or truthfulness of confessions. It focuses only on capacities to have provided knowing, intelligent, and voluntary waivers of *Miranda* rights.

This book will not focus on the second context DeClue identified—evaluating risk factors that might be associated with a coerced confession. Such an evaluation would involve the assessment of the circumstances under which the

INFO

DeClue (2005) identified three ways in which a mental health professional may conduct an evaluation of voluntariness. The evaluator may be called on to:

1. assess the validity of a Miranda waiver

2. evaluate factors that may have contributed to a coerced confession

3. evaluate the truthfulness of a confession

confession was offered (the situational characteristics of the interrogation) and/or the characteristics of the defendant that might have contributed to susceptibility to coercion. Experts can present information to the court about how these factors *might* have contributed to a coerced confession. Although these characteristics may or may not be related to capacities to have waived rights, this forensic question is distinct from questions about the validity of a *Miranda* waiver. In addition, assessment of factors that could have contributed to false confessions is a legitimate area of psycho-legal evaluation. However, a discussion of such methodology would be inappropriate in a book on "best practices." Evaluation of factors that could have affected the veracity of confessions is a field of study for which "best practice" standards do not exist. Consequently, presentation of such methodology would reflect the personal opinions and preferences of the authors rather than a widely accepted, empirically based standard of practice. Thus, evaluation practices presented in this book are limited to established methods that focus on assessing those capacities directly related to the legal requirements for providing a valid *Miranda* waiver.

With regard to the third context in which voluntariness may be at issue, the authors of this book agree with DeClue (2005). No expert can offer an opinion about whether or not a confession was, in fact, truthful. The authors of this book and the editors of this series believe that, at the present time, there is no established standard of practice in forensic psychology for evaluating the factual accuracy of a defendant's confession. Similarly, the authors of this book, along with the series editors, are unaware of any published research that has reviewed how forensic mental health experts approach these evaluations; in other words, there is no established consensus about how these evaluations are or should be conducted.

In sum, this book focuses exclusively on evaluations of the validity of *Miranda* waivers and factors associated with increased likelihood of suspects providing waivers that did not meet the knowing, intelligent, and voluntary requirements established by case law. A comprehensive consideration of risk factors related to coerced and false confessions can be found in Gudjonsson (1992),

Wrightman and Kassin (1993), Shuy (1998), White (2001), Oberlander, Goldstein, and Goldstein (2003), DeClue (2005), Kassin (2005), Leo (2008), Kassin (in press), and Kassin et al. (2010).

How Often Is the Legal Validity of *Miranda* Waivers Raised as an Issue in Court?

Little data are available about the frequency with which attorneys challenge the admissibility of confessions based on invalid *Miranda* waivers. However, we do know that about 80% of suspects waive the rights to silence and counsel (Cassell & Hayman, 1996; Leo, 1996), and the majority of suspects offer self-incriminating statements when questioned by police (Pearse & Gudjonsson, 1997). Adult suspects waive their rights at high rates, but juveniles, individuals with mental retardation, and individuals with mental illness waive their rights even more frequently and have characteristics that put them at risk for failing to understand and appreciate their *Miranda* rights and voluntarily waive these rights. See chapter 3 for a summary of the available literature on the frequency of *Miranda* waivers and legal challenges to the resulting confessions.

Legal Standards

Miranda v. Arizona specified those rights guaranteed by the Constitution and established the legal standard by which a defendant can validly waive those rights. In fact, *Miranda* rights are thought to be so familiar that, in 2000, Chief Justice Rehnquist wrote that they have become "embedded in routine police practice to the point where the warnings have become part of our national culture" (*Dickerson v. United States*)." Despite the landmark nature of the *Miranda* decision, earlier cases acknowledged the right of defendants to exercise the Constitutional protections of

INFO

Juveniles, mentally retarded individuals, and persons who suffer from mental illness are more likely than other individuals to waive their Miranda rights without fully understanding and appreciating them.

silence and legal counsel. As such, *Miranda* rights evolved some-what gradually over a number of decades.

Pre-*Miranda* Decisions

Prior to *Miranda v. Arizona*, the U.S. Supreme Court decided a range of cases that established the limits of acceptable police practices when conducting interrogations. DeClue (2005) reviewed many of these cases, some of which are cited in this volume. A common theme reflected in many of the Court's holdings was an attempt to balance the law enforcement's need to function effectively and obtain information about a crime with the Constitutional protection of citizens' rights—"Our Constitution, unlike some others, strikes a balance in favor of the right of the accused to be advised by his lawyer of his privilege against self-incrimination" (*Escobedo v. Illinois*, 1964). These pre-*Miranda* decisions typically focused on the voluntariness of confessions, often linking unconstitutional police interrogation practices with an increased likelihood of false confessions.

BROWN V. MISSISSIPPI (1936)

At a murder trial, police officers testified that, when initially interrogated, an African American defendant accused of murder denied his involvement in the crime. The U.S. Supreme Court reviewed further trial testimony: "[T]hey had seized him, and with participation of the deputy they hanged him by a rope to the limb of a tree, and having let him down, they hung him again, and when he was let down the second time, and he still protested his innocence, he was tried to a tree and whipped, and still declining to accede to the demands that he confess, he was finally released. . . . [The next day he was] again severely whipped . . . and the defendant then agreed to confess." The defendant, along with two other codefendants, had his sentence vacated by the Court. The Court held that these interrogation techniques, involving

CASE LAW

Brown v.
Mississippi
(1936)

● The Court held that brutal and violent interrogation techniques used to coerce a confession violate due process and cannot be entered as evidence.

"brutality and violence" to coerce a confession, violated the Fourteenth Amendment. The Court opined, "the rack and the torture chamber may not be substituted for the witness stand." This case clearly indicated that confessions could not be coerced by physical threat, intimidation, or brutality.

SPANO V. NEW YORK (1959)

In *Spano*, the Court "extended the concept of coercion to include not only physical brutality, but psychological pressure as well" (Oberlander, Goldstein, & Goldstein, 2003, p. 336). The plaintiff, with no criminal record, was accused of the murder of a former boxer, someone who had beaten and robbed him. Allegedly, Spano confronted his assailant and shot him. When questioned by interrogators, Spano denied the murder, but, after eight hours of questioning by a number of interrogators, he confessed. In its decision, the Court noted the petitioner's history of emotional instability; his intellectual limitations (he had been rejected by the military for having failed an intelligence test); the length of the interrogation ("until almost sunrise"); his ignored requests to contact his attorney; and the participation of a childhood acquaintance in the questioning, someone who was preparing to be a police officer. The Court concluded "that petitioner's will was overborne by official pressure, fatigue and sympathy falsely aroused, after considering all the facts in their post-indictment setting." The Court acknowledged that there is a conflict between the need for effective, prompt law enforcement and the importance of protecting citizens from "unconstitutional methods of law enforcement . . . in the end life and liberty can be as much endangered from illegal methods used to convict those thought to be criminals as from the actual criminals themselves."

ESCOBEDO V. ILLINOIS (1964)

Escobedo, along with his sister, was accused of the murder of his brother-in-law. Officers testified that Escobedo, who initially denied his role in the crime, was not formally

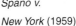

CASE LAW

Spano v.
New York (1959)

● The Court ruled that coercion is not limited only to physical violence and brutality, but psychological pressure as well.

charged but was in custody and was not free to leave. He had retained an attorney prior to the start of the interrogation, but when the lawyer arrived at the Detective Bureau, the attorney was told that the police were still questioning his client. Escobedo testified that he had repeatedly asked to see his lawyer but was informed that his lawyer "did not want to see him." The Court found that during the course of questioning, no one had advised the plaintiff of his Constitutional rights, including "informing him of his absolute right to remain silent. . . . " As such, the Court held that this omission was "offensive to fairness and equity," and "The right to counsel would indeed be hollow if it began at a period when few confessions are obtained." In a strongly worded decision, the Court stated, "No system of criminal justice can, or should, survive if it comes to depend for its continued effectiveness on the citizens' abdication through unawareness of their constitutional rights."

KENT V. UNITED STATES (1966)

Kent was decided by the U.S. Supreme Court less than three months before its *Miranda* decision. The plaintiff, Morris Kent, was convicted of housebreaking and robbery, crimes committed when he was 16 years old. He had been questioned by police officers and admitted his involvement in this and other crimes. Kent was transferred from juvenile court to adult court without benefit of a hearing and was tried as an adult. The Court focused its decision on "the justifiability of affording less protection than is accorded to adults suspected of criminal offenses. . . . " In the majority opinion, Justice Fortas wrote, "the child receives the worst of both worlds: that he gets neither the protections accorded to adults nor the solicitous care and regenerative treatment postulated for children." Although the court side-stepped issues focusing on the rights that might be afforded to juveniles other than a hearing on the transfer to adult court, the decision emphasized, "Under our Constitution, the condition of being a boy does not justify a kangaroo court." Less than three months later, in

Miranda, the Court would spell out the rights to which adult suspects were entitled and, one year later, the Court would extend those same rights to juveniles in the case of *In re Gault* (1967).

MIRANDA V. ARIZONA (1966)

The previous cases set the stage for *Miranda v. Arizona*. The *Miranda* decision reflected the Court's increasing concern that suspects, under the pressure of police interrogation, would be vulnerable to purposeful or inadvertent denials of their Constitutional rights to silence and legal counsel; the Court was, therefore, concerned that suspects would offer incriminating statements about crimes they may not have committed.

The *Miranda* decision addressed four separate cases that came before the Court in 1966 (*Miranda v. Arizona* [Docket No. 759], *Vignera v. New York* [Docket No. 760], *Westover v. United States* [Docket No. 761], and *California v. Stewart* [Docket No. 584]). In a 5–4 majority opinion authored by Chief Justice Warren, the Court noted that the fact pattern in all four cases was similar. The defendants were in police custody; they were interrogated as criminal suspects for the purpose of obtaining confessions; they were "cut off from the outside world," "incommunicado"; they found themselves in a "police-dominated atmosphere"; they all denied committing the criminal acts; they were interrogated for a number of hours; and they all eventually provided confessions. In addition, police misconduct was *not* alleged in any of these cases. The decision emphasized, "the modern practice of in-custody interrogation is psychological rather than physically oriented." Further, the Court stated, "the blood of the accused is not the only hallmark of an unconstitutional inquisition."

In the lead case, the plaintiff, Ernesto Miranda, had been arrested and charged with kidnapping and rape. He was brought to a Phoenix police station, identified by a

CASE LAW

Kent v. United States (1966)

- The Court held that certain due process protections, in this case a hearing on the transfer of the case from juvenile court to adult court, were required in juvenile court proceedings.

witness, and taken into an interrogation room. Miranda initially denied involvement in this crime, but confessed following a two-hour interrogation. At the top of his written statement was a paragraph indicating that his "confession was made voluntarily, without threats or promises of immunity and 'with full knowledge of my legal rights, understanding any statement I make may be used against me'." At his trial, police officers testified, "Miranda was not advised that he had a right to have an attorney present." His confession was admitted into evidence over the objections of his attorney, and he was convicted and sentenced to 20 to 30 years imprisonment on each count. The Arizona Supreme Court held, on appeal, that his rights were not violated, affirming his conviction. They emphasized that he had not "specifically requested counsel" (*Miranda v. Arizona*).

The U.S. Supreme Court reversed Miranda's conviction, stating, "From the testimony of the officers and by the admission of the respondent, it is clear that Miranda was not in any way apprised of his right to consult with an attorney and to have one present during the interrogation, nor was his right not to be compelled to incriminate himself effectively protected in any manner." The Court emphasized the pressure inherent in custodial interrogations, including quotes from commonly-used interrogation manuals (i.e., Inbau & Reid, 1962) to demonstrate defendants' disadvantage when confronted by trained interrogators. To "level the playing field," the Court indicated, suspects should be reminded of their Constitutional rights. Without attributing misconduct to the interrogators in any of the four cases, the Court stated, "The very fact of custodial interrogation exacts a heavy toll on individual liberty and trades on the weakness of individuals." As such, the Court acknowledged that interrogators had failed to provide adequate "safeguards at the outset of the interrogation to insure that the statements were truly the product of free choice." Miranda's conviction was reversed. Ironically, Miranda was stabbed to death in a bar fight years later. He had earned money autographing cards with the warnings that bear his name.

In order "to protect precious Fifth Amendment rights" the Court ruled that, to "scrupulously honor" the right against self-incrimination, a suspect taken into custody must be warned before questioning that:

> . . . he has the right to remain silent, that anything he says can be used against him in a court of law, that he has the right to the presence of an attorney, and that if he can't afford an attorney one will be appointed for him prior to any questioning if he so desires (p. 479).

Miranda does not prohibit police from questioning suspects. People can be questioned without being given the warnings when in community settings; they can be asked semi-formal questions in their homes; they can be questioned following traffic stops; they can give unwarned statements during the booking process; statements can be obtained without the warnings if the public's safety is at risk; and suspects can be questioned in police cars on the way to more formal interrogation settings (see Melton et al., 2007 for a review of case law in which courts have determined that confessions, under specific circumstances, may be admissible if given without prior administration of the *Miranda* warning). Promises and inducements made by police prior to obtaining a confession may be legally permissible if the suspect has not been explicitly told that the confession would aid the defense or that it would result in a lesser sentence (*Commonwealth v. Meehan*, 1979; *Commonwealth v. Mandile*, 1986). Despite these conclusions in decisions on admissibility, court rulings have been inconsistent on the legality of various police interrogation tactics to encourage confessions (Oberlander, Goldstein, & Goldstein, 2003).

Despite the variability in decisions about what should constitute a custodial interrogation that would require the administration of warnings, the Supreme Court was very clear that the Constitutional guarantees to silence and counsel in custodial interrogation can only be waived *knowingly*, *intelligently*, and *voluntarily*. Furthermore, it ruled that even though a defendant may have signed a

INFO

Miranda does not universally prohibit police from questioning subjects without warning. For example, people can be questioned without warning in community settings, during traffic stops, and when the public's safety is at risk.

"clause stating that he had full knowledge of his legal rights [this acknowledgment] did not approach [the] knowing and intelligent waiver required to relinquish [the] constitutional rights to counsel and privilege against self-incrimination." In *Miranda*, the Court emphasized the significance of the requirement that the waiver be valid; "This Court has always set high standards of proof for the waiver of constitutional rights, and we reassert these standards as applied to in-custody interrogation."

"Knowing" as a legal concept

Although the "knowing" and "intelligent" requirements were specified in the *Miranda* decision, the Court did not define these terms. Rather, individual states were left to develop their own legal definitions of these constructs required by the Court for a valid rights waiver.

Regarding the knowing requirement, Grisso (1981, 2003) emphasized, "No particular degree of capacity to understand these rights and entitlements necessarily satisfies the 'knowing' component" (Grisso, 2003, p. 151). Melton et al. (2007) defined "knowing" with the question, "did the defendant understand that he or she was waiving rights...?" (p. 171). Courts consider the "*totality of circumstances*" in determining whether an individual defendant understood her rights at the time of her waiver. This approach, to be discussed from a legal perspective later in this chapter and from a psychological/psychiatric perspective in chapter 2, requires the judge to consider an almost unlimited range of variables, including characteristics of both the defendant (i.e., age, intelligence, prior experience with the police) and the interrogative situation (i.e., number of interrogators, size of the interrogation room, length of the interrogation), when reaching a decision about the validity of a waiver.

A federal court's decision in *Coyote v. United States* (1967) offers a somewhat simple perspective on the meaning of "knowing": "*Miranda* requires meaningful advice to the unlettered and unlearned in language which he can comprehend and on which he can knowingly act. . . ." In *People v. Lara* (1967), the court indicated that adolescents might have difficulty "fully comprehending the meaning of the effect of the waiver." Similarly, in

West v. United States (1968) and *Fare v. Michael C.* (1979), courts recognized that juveniles might be at a disadvantage in their abilities to understand their rights because of deficits in intelligence and functioning (see Feld, 2000; Grisso, 1998). In *United States ex rel. Simon v. Maroney* (1964), the court ruled the confession inadmissible based on the defendant's lack of capacity to understand the meaning of the waiver. In *In re Patrick W.* (1978), the court opined, "the courts have always given more zealous protection to minors' rights, under both criminal law and civil, because of their relative helplessness when dealing with adults by reason of immaturity." Similarly, *People v. Higgins* (1993) required police interrogators to "do something more" than merely provide a rote reading and explanation of the *Miranda* rights prior to questioning suspects when they have reason to believe that the suspects may have difficulty understanding their rights. "Special populations include children and adolescents, individuals with mental illness, those with mental deficiencies, and individuals with organic impairment" (Oberlander, Goldstein, & Goldstein, 2003, p. 339). Grisso (2003) concluded, "legal standards usually construe 'knowing' as a sum of the suspects' ability to understand plus the manner in which they are informed [of their rights]" (p. 151). Chapter 2 describes "knowing" in psycho-legal terms and considers it from a forensic mental health perspective.

"Intelligent" as a legal concept

Grisso (2003) distinguished between the "knowing" and "intelligent" requirements for a legally valid waiver of *Miranda* rights: "a suspect may *understand* that she has a right to speak with an attorney, as the *Miranda* warnings indicate; but she might not *grasp the significance* of being able to speak with an attorney (for example, might not know what an attorney is or does) and therefore be unable to 'intelligently' decide to claim or waive the right" (p. 152). Citing Grisso (2003), Frumkin (2008) distinguished an intelligent from a knowing waiver by focusing on the defendant's "decision-making capacity, whereby the subject weighs options and his or her consequences" (p. 138). A definition of "intelligent," was provided by Melton and colleagues (2007) to forensic mental health evaluators in the form of a question: "was the waiver of rights the product of rational reasoning process?" (p. 171). In chapter 2, we operationalize "intelligent" as a forensic mental health concept that can be assessed.

A review of case law reveals some disagreement about the depth of comprehension required for a valid rights waiver. For example, in *People v. Williams* (1984) and *People v. Bernasco* (1990), the courts ruled that a valid waiver did not require understanding of the underlying legal reasons behind each right. *Williams* required only that the suspect grasp the immediate import of the warnings. That is, the suspect need not grasp the pros and cons associated with waiving the rights and understand or provide an accurate definition of the word "right." The court held that suspects did not need to possess or be provided with a legal education by interrogators or prosecutors. Similarly, *Bernasco* stated that it is not necessary that suspects have "the ability to understand far-reaching legal and strategic effects of waiving one's rights or to appreciate how widely or deeply an interrogation may probe. . . . If intelligent knowledge [a term that fuses two of the *Miranda* requirements] in the *Miranda* context means anything, it means the ability to understand the very words used in the warnings."

In contrast to the simplistic level of knowledge required in these two cases, other cases (e.g., *Coyote v. United States; People v. Baker*, 1973; *People v. Lara*, 1967) required deeper comprehension of rights for a waiver to be legally valid. Most notably, these cases required more than mere linguistic comprehension; they also required that the suspect grasp the concept of a "right" as protected and recognize the advantages of having legal representation before agreeing to speak with interrogators. For instance, *People v. Lara* required a showing that a defendant "fully comprehend the meaning and effect" of the warnings. *In re Patrick W.* viewed the defendant as having provided an "intelligent" waiver if he had the ability to "fully comprehend the meaning and effect of his decision to waive the rights and make incriminating statements to the police officers." In *Moran v. Burbine* (1986), the Court held that "the waiver must have been made with a full awareness of both the nature of the right being abandoned and the consequences of the decision to abandon it."

In reviewing case law on the "intelligent" requirement, Grisso (2003) concluded, "it is unclear what the law intends when it refers to an 'intelligent' waiver of rights, or whether the term has any meaning separate from 'understanding'" (p. 152). Frumkin (2008) emphatically stated, "An unintelligent waiver does not have to do with making a poor choice. An unintelligent waiver results from making a decision to waive the rights based on a misunderstanding of the legal process and how it applies both personally and in the abstract" (p. 139). In considering the contradictions that appear in case law from state to state, it is clear that the expert must be familiar with the "depth" of comprehension that is legally required for the "intelligent" requirement to be met.

"Voluntary" as a legal concept

In *Miranda*, the Court addressed the issue of voluntary waivers: "Whatever the testimony of the authorities as to the waiver of rights by the accused, the fact of lengthy interrogation or incommunicado incarceration before the statement is made is strong evidence that the accused did not validly waive his rights." The Court emphasized the need to consider "the compelling influence of the interrogation" as a factor that "finally forced" the suspect to confess. Similarly, evidence "that the accused was threatened, tricked, or cajoled into a waiver, will, of course, show that the defendant did not voluntarily waive his privilege." In *Moran v. Burbine*, the U.S. Supreme Court noted that rights must be waived voluntarily "in the sense that it was the product of a free and deliberate choice rather than intimidation, coercion, or deception."

Grisso (2003) observed that the voluntary prong of *Miranda* "requires that the waiver decision must be a consequence of the suspect's free will, rather that a product of coercion" (p. 153). Melton and colleagues (2007) described voluntariness with the question, "was the situation in its totality—and in its interaction with the defendant's state of mind—so coercive that the defendant's will was overborne?" (p. 171). DeClue (2005) and Oberlander, Goldstein, and Goldstein (2003) emphasized that, when considering conducting forensic mental health assessment of voluntariness, evaluators should focus on whether police behavior was coercive, as this practice reflects the legal requirements for a valid waiver. Again, judges consider characteristics of both the defendant and the interrogation to determine whether police took advantage of these characteristics to obtain an involuntary waiver of rights.

Colorado v. Connelly (1986) further clarified the concept of voluntariness. In this unusual case, the suspect fled to Denver from Boston, walked up to a police officer, and reported that he wanted to confess to a murder. The officer immediately administered the *Miranda* rights, and Connelly, then, offered a confession to a murder he had committed months before. The confession was introduced at trial, and Connelly was convicted. An appeal to the U.S. Supreme Court was based, in part, on Connelly's claim that the confession had been coerced, not by the police, but by his own command auditory hallucinations (the voice of God). The Court ruled that coercion must be a product of police misconduct and that when an individual confesses because of command auditory hallucinations, he has chosen to do so. The Court held that without evidence of coercive police conduct causally related to the confession, there is no basis to conclude that the defendant was deprived of his due process rights. Melton et al. (2007). In other words, a finding of involuntariness must arise from police misconduct. Forensic mental health experts in such cases must focus on the ways in which possible police misconduct during interrogation interacted with suspect and interrogative characteristics to result in an involuntary waiver of rights.

Post-*Miranda* Cases

Following the *Miranda* decision in 1966, a range of legal questions emerged about the proper administration of these rights. Among the issues considered by the U.S. Supreme Court were the application of *Miranda* rights to juvenile offenders; the range of circumstances a judge should consider when ruling whether the rights in a specific case were validly waived; what should happen when a defendant provides an invalid confession initially (i.e., without having been appropriately administered the *Miranda* warning) and then provides a second confession after the warnings are administered; and whether an act of Congress can override the Court's *Miranda* decision. There are hundreds of relevant appeal court decisions and numerous U.S. Supreme Court decisions that have been issued post-*Miranda*. A thorough review of many of these cases can be found in DeClue (2005) and Melton et al. (2007).

IN RE GAULT (1967)

Gerald Gault was 15 years old when he was picked up by the police from his parents' home while they were at work. He was taken into custody, brought to the police station, charged with having made a lewd telephone call, and questioned by a police officer. Gault's parents were not informed that he had been arrested. He was given a hearing in juvenile court the following afternoon, but no transcript was made of the hearing. Gault testified, although there is disagreement about whether he admitted to the alleged offense during that hearing.

Consistent with the Arizona Juvenile Code, Gault was denied due process rights afforded to adults. Gault was not provided with a notice of the charges against him; the complainant was not present at the hearing and, as such, he could not be cross-examined; neither Gault nor his parents were provided with timely notice of the hearing; Gault was not provided with a lawyer and he was never told that he had a right to legal representation. He was never informed of a right against self-incrimination, told that he did not have to make statement, or informed that what he said might lead to his classification as a "delinquent." During his hearing, the juvenile court judge questioned him, a process followed at a second hearing as well. Again, because of the lack of transcripts, it is unclear what Gault said, if anything.

Gault was committed to a state industrial school for up to six years—until he reached the age of majority in Arizona. Unlike adults convicted of a crime, Gault did not have the right to appeal this decision. Furthermore, had Gault been an adult whose case was decided in adult court, the maximum penalty would have been a fine of $5 to $10 *or* imprisonment for up to two months.

The U.S. Supreme Court agreed to hear Gault's case. The state had argued that because Gault was tried as a juvenile, he was not entitled to the due process rights granted to adults. The state's argument emphasized that youth are not punished, but instead receive rehabilitation and appropriate treatment within the juvenile justice system. However, in a 7 to 2 decision, writing for the majority, Justice Fortas emphatically rejected this notion. The Court noted that when a juvenile is placed in a detention facility "freedom is curtailed." The Court held, "unbridled discretion, however benevolently motivated, is frequently a poor substitute for principle and procedure." In *Gault*, the Court opined, "Instead of mother and father and brothers and friends and classmates, his world is peopled by guards, custodians, state employees, and 'delinquents' confined with him for anything from waywardness to rape and homicide." In its decision, the Court held, "neither the Fourteenth Amendment nor the Bill of Rights is for adults only."

In discussing the *Gault* decision, Melton and colleagues (2007) referred to it as "doubtless the most important case in juvenile law specifically and children's rights generally" (p. 467). The deprivation of civil rights, common in juvenile courts throughout the country ended, as the Court declared, "the condition of being a boy does not justify a kangaroo court." The *Gault* Court indicated that, for juveniles, confessions should not be "a product of ignorance of rights or of adolescent fantasy, fright or despair." In essence, the Court held that the privilege against self-incrimination is a safeguard against confessions being obtained "by force or by psychological domination." Consequently, Gault extended all rights (with the exception of trial by a jury of peers) afforded to adults

CASE LAW

In re Gault

(1967)

- A landmark U.S. Supreme Court decision which established that under the Fourteenth Amendment, juveniles accused of crimes in a delinquency proceeding must be accorded the same due process rights as adults.

in criminal court to juveniles, regardless of whether their cases are heard in juvenile or criminal court. This set of rights includes the requirement that the *Miranda* warnings be administered to juveniles prior to police interrogation in custodial settings.

COYOTE V. UNITED STATES (1967)

Willie Salt Coyote was arrested in New Mexico, driving a pickup truck stolen earlier that day in Colorado. He was taken to a New Mexico police station, and an FBI agent introduced himself and read Coyote his *Miranda* rights. The appellant indicated that he understood his rights, but explained that he was sleepy and had been drinking. He was given coffee and then permitted to sleep. When awakened about one hour later, Coyote was again administered his rights and acknowledged that he understood them. Interrogation began, and Coyote provided a statement in which he admitted to the crime. When the FBI agent began to type the statement, Coyote offered to type it himself, explaining that he had attended a business college and was a skilled typist. Nonetheless, the agent completed the typed statement, which included a section that acknowledged, "I have also been told by Special Agent Jackson that I can talk to a lawyer or anyone before saying anything, and that the judge will get me a lawyer if I am broke." Coyote signed the statement.

Coyote was tried, convicted, and sentenced to five years imprisonment. He appealed his conviction on a number of grounds, including the claim that he did not understand that he could have a lawyer appointed *before* going to court. His claim focused on the wording of the warning cited above. In summary, the court wrote that his appeal "reflects that appellant was not informed with sufficient clarity of his right to a court appointed attorney at the time the statement was made. . . . Specifically he says that the comma preceding the phrase 'and the judge will get me a lawyer if I am broke' renders the sentence susceptible of the interpretation [sic] that court appointed counsel would be available only after appellant had been before the judge."

In rejecting Coyote's appeal, the court stated, "We will not indulge semantic debates between counsel over the particular words used to inform an individual of his rights. The crucial test is whether the words in the context used, considering the age, background and intelligence of the individual being interrogated, impart a clear understandable warning of all of his rights." The court also noted that after he was arrested, there was little delay in reading Coyote his rights. He was not "denied food, drink and sleep, or promised leniency. . . . " The role of the court in considering issues related to the validity of *Miranda* waivers involves, "objectively determining whether in the *circumstances of the case* the words used were sufficient to convey the required warnings [emphasis added]." In effect, the court advanced the concept that legal decisions must be based on a consideration of the *totality of circumstances* surrounding the presentation of rights, the interrogation process, and factors specific to the defendant—each on a case by case basis.

The *totality of circumstances* approach was extended to juveniles 12 years later in *Fare v. Michael C.* (1979). These cases, along with *Johnson v. Zerbst* (1938) and *West v. United States* (1968), provided a list of factors to be considered within the *totality of circumstances* test, including the suspect's age, intelligence, education, literacy and language ability, prior experience with the police and courts, mental health, conduct, maturity, and vulnerability, as well as the physical conditions of the interrogation, and whether the suspect was held incommunicado prior to police questioning (DeClue, 2005; Frumkin, 2000; Grisso, 1998, 2003; Oberlander, 1998; Oberlander & Goldstein, 2001; Oberlander, Goldstein, & Goldstein, 2003). The forensic mental health perspective on the *totality of circumstances* is reviewed in the following two chapters, along with the extant research on the relationships between the *totality of circumstances* factors and capacity to waive rights.

CASE LAW

Coyote v.
United States
(1967)

- The Court advanced the concept that legal decisions must be based on a consideration of the totality of circumstances.

- The Court provided a list of factors (defendant characteristics and physical conditions of the interrogation) to be considered within the totality of circumstances test.

FARE V. MICHAEL C. (1979)

Michael C. was 16 ½ years old when taken into police custody, suspected of committing murder while robbing the victim's home. He had a number of prior arrests and had been on probation since he was 12 years old. Michael C. was administered his *Miranda* rights prior to interrogation, and he was questioned by two police officers who taped their conversation with him. When he was asked, "Do you want to give up your right to have an attorney present here while we talk?" he asked, "Can I have my probation officer here?" He was told, "[We] can't get a hold of your probation officer right now. You have the right to an attorney." Michael C. then agreed to speak to the interrogators, drew sketches of the crime scene, and provided a statement implicating himself in the crime. He was found guilty of the charges and appealed, claiming that his request to speak with his probation officer was tantamount to asking for an attorney. The California Supreme Court held that his request for his probation officer was a *per se* equivalent of his invocation of his Fifth Amendment right, as delineated in *Miranda*. In essence, they held that no factors other than this juvenile's request to speak to an attorney needed to be considered by the court to conclude that he had been deprived of his constitutional rights. The U. S. Supreme Court considered this decision.

Justice Blackmun wrote the majority opinion for the Court. He indicated, "the lawyer occupies a critical position over the legal system because of his unique ability to protect the Fifth Amendment right of a client undergoing custodial interrogation." The Court noted that a probation office is not trained in the law and is an employee of the state. A probation officer has the responsibility to take a youth into custody if he is suspected of violating terms of his parole or breaks the law. The Court pointed out that it was, in fact, Michael C.'s probation officer who had filed the complaint against him in this case. The decision indicated that the court needed to consider the totality of the circumstances surrounding the interrogation to determine if the *Miranda* rights had been validly waived. The Court, therefore, adopted the same totality of circumstance test required by judges to rule on the validity of adults' waivers, as established in *West v. United States, People v. Lara,* and *Coyote v. United States.*

The Court rejected the California appeals court's decision that Michael C.'s request to speak to his probation officer was, per se, a reason to exclude his inculpatory statement. They stated, "we decline to attach such overwhelming significance to this request." Factors that comprised the *totality of circumstances* in this landmark decision included the "juvenile's age, experience, education, background, and intelligence and . . . whether he has the capacity to understand the warnings given to him, the nature of the Fifth Amendment, and the rights, and the consequences of those rights." In rejecting the California appeals court's reasoning (and consistent with the *totality of circumstances* perspective that would now apply to juveniles), it was noted that Michael C. had considerable experience with the juvenile justice system, including a number of arrests, a sentence at a youth camp, and years of probation. He had not been tricked or "worn down" by interrogators, interrogation was not prolonged, and he was neither threatened nor intimidated by the police.

In a highly critical analysis of this legal decision, Feld (2000) commented that the Court rejected "developmental or psychological differences between juveniles and adults" (p. 112). He stated that the case incorrectly "affirms adolescents' ability to make autonomous legal decisions without additional special procedures, and enables police interrogators to take advantage of their manifest social-psychological limitations relative to adults" (p. 112). In chapter 3 of this volume, we discuss the potential impact of cognitive, developmental, and neurological immaturity on capacities to validly waive rights.

CASE LAW
Fare v.
Michael C.
(1979)

● The Court held that the Miranda rule is based on the unique role the lawyer plays in the adversary system of criminal justice.

DICKERSON V. UNITED STATES (2000)

Shortly after the *Miranda* decision, the U.S. Congress attempted to overrule *Miranda* through legislation (18 U.S.C. 3501)—no longer would *Miranda* warnings be required in federal cases. The only prerequisite for admission of a confession would be that it was voluntarily given. The law, which was passed in 1968, instructed judges to consider, on a case-by-case basis, the *totality of circumstances* under which a confession had been obtained to determine the voluntariness of the confession. In effect, this "law essentially returned interrogation procedures to the pre-*Miranda* era. . . . Because of the relationship between the legislative powers of Congress and the judicial powers of the Supreme Court, the new law could be upheld only if successful legal challenges were made to *Miranda*" (Oberlander, Goldstein, & Goldstein, 2003, p. 337). This law was upheld in federal court in *United States v. Crocker* (1975), but largely ignored in federal cases, and *Miranda* rights continued to be administered. The law was challenged in *Dickerson v. United States* (2000).

In *Dickerson*, the petitioner moved to suppress statements he had made to an FBI agent about his involvement in a bank robbery and other federal crimes. He claimed that police did not administer the *Miranda* warnings prior to interrogation. Although his motion was granted by the federal District Court, it was denied by the Circuit Court of Appeals because, under Rule 3501, his statement had been obtained voluntarily. Writing for the 7 to 2 majority, Chief Justice Rehnquist stated, in a strongly worded decision, "*Miranda*, being a constitutional decision of the court, may not be in effect overruled by an Act of Congress. . . . " The majority opinion stated, "Whether or not we would agree with *Miranda*'s reasoning and its resulting rule, were we addressing the issue in the first instance, the principles of *stare decisis* weigh heavily against overruling it now." This principle, to let stand that which was previously decided, influenced the Court in its deference to *Miranda*. The Court also noted in *Dickerson* that *Miranda* warnings had "become embedded in routine police practice to the point where the warnings have become part of our national culture." The Court declared

CASE LAW

Dickerson v.
United States
(2000)

● The U.S. Supreme
Court upheld the
requirement that the
Miranda warning be
read to criminal
suspects.

18 U.S.C. 3501 unconstitutional, stating, "*Miranda* requires procedures that will warn a suspect in custody of his right to remain silent which will assure the suspect that the exercise of that right will be honored." As such, *Dickerson v. United States* affirmed the importance of *Miranda* to the justice system.

FELLERS V. UNITED STATES (2004) AND *MISSOURI V. SIEBERT* (2004)

Both of these cases have similar fact patterns and raise a similar legal question. What is the admissibility of a confession given after police administered the *Miranda* rights but that followed an earlier statement that had not been preceded by *Miranda* warnings? In each case, police interrogated the suspect without first providing the warnings required under *Miranda*. After confessing to the crime, a brief time period elapsed, and the suspect was then fully informed of his constitutional rights. At this point, Fellers and Siebert both waived their rights and confessed to the crimes for a second time.

In the first case, Fellers moved to have both admissions suppressed. Following a hearing, the Magistrate Judge excluded the first confession in its entirety, and also excluded portions of the second confession as "fruits of the prior failure to provide *Miranda* warnings." However, upon appeal, although the court supported exclusion of the unwarned statement, it ruled the second statement admissible. The Court of Appeals ruled that Fellers had waived his rights knowingly and voluntarily, citing *Oregon v. Elstad* (1985), a case indicating that if a defendant had waived *Miranda* rights knowingly and voluntarily before offering a confession, the statements should be considered constitutionally obtained. Fellers was convicted at trial and appealed, arguing that the second statement was fruit of the unwarned confession he had provided earlier.

In *Fellers v. United States* (2004), the U.S. Supreme Court indicated that the petitioner had been questioned "deliberately and designedly . . . to elicit information [about a crime]." Fellers had not been given the opportunity to have a lawyer, a violation of the Sixth Amendment. In its decision, the Court cited an earlier case, *United States v. Wade* (1967), which established the right of a defendant to a lawyer in a post-indictment lineup, even if Fifth Amendment rights are not yet relevant. In a unanimous opinion about the *Fellers* case, Justice O'Connor wrote that the admissibility of the second confession, obtained after rights were waived, did not "turn solely on whether the statements were 'knowingly and voluntarily made.'" Rather, the Court held, "We have not had occasion to decide whether the rationale of *Elstad* applies when a suspect makes incriminating statements after a knowing and voluntary waiver of his right to counsel notwithstanding earlier police questioning in violation of Sixth Amendment standards. We therefore remand to the Court of Appeals to address this issue in the first instance." As such, the Court did not offer an opinion on what should be done with a Mirandized confession that follows an un-Mirandized one.

Approximately five months later, in *Missouri v. Siebert* (2004), the Court pointedly addressed the question it had side-stepped in *Fellers*—what should be done with a Mirandized confession that follows a statement given under circumstances in which *Miranda* rights should have been administered but were not? In *Siebert*, the Petitioner, Patrice Siebert, had been questioned about a fire that she had started in her mobile home. Her 12-year-old son, suffering from cerebral palsy, had died in his sleep. Fearing that she would be charged with neglect, she started the fire to cover up his death. She was questioned for 30 to 40 minutes at a police station days after the fire, and provided a confession. The interrogator admitted that he had made a conscious decision not to advise her of her rights. Following a 20-minute coffee and cigarette break, the interrogator returned, and read her the *Miranda* rights; she signed the waiver and, then, offered a second confession.

The District Court suppressed the first confession, but it allowed the second confession, which followed administration of the *Miranda* warning, to be entered into evidence. Siebert was convicted of second degree murder and appealed her conviction, arguing that the second confession should have been excluded from trial under the "fruit of the poisonous tree" doctrine. The Missouri Court of Appeals held that, under *Oregon v. Elstad* (1985), "a suspect's unwarned inculpatory statement made during a brief exchange at his house did not make a later, fully warned inculpatory statement inadmissible." However, the Missouri State Supreme Court held that Siebert's Mirandized statement should be suppressed as well because it was given nearly continuously with the first admission.

In a 5 to 4 plurality decision (i.e., two concurring opinions were written), the U.S. Supreme Court affirmed the Missouri Supreme Court's decision. Justice Souter wrote, "By any objective measure, it is likely that warnings withheld until after interrogation and confession will be ineffective in preparing a suspect for successive interrogation, close in time and similar in content . . . it would be unrealistic to treat two spates of integrated and proximately conducted questioning as independent interrogations, subject to independent evaluation simply because *Miranda* warnings formally punctuated them in the middle." The Court clearly indicated that, under such circumstances, "a reasonable person in the suspect's shoes could not have understood . . . that she retained a choice about continuing to talk." As a potential solution to the dilemma faced by interrogators in such cases, Justice Souter proposed that "a substantial break in time and circumstances" be taken between the time the unwarned confession was given and the readings of the *Miranda* rights prior to the second interrogation. Similarly, Justice Breyer, in his concurring opinion, wrote that under such circumstances, an effective *Miranda* warning can be given, "only when certain circumstances—a lapse in time, a change in location or interrogating officer, or a shift in the focus of the questioning—intervene between the unwarned questioning and any postwarning statement."

A major problem arises when forensic mental health experts encounter cases involving pre- and post-warning confessions. How much time is required for the effects of the first confession to "attenuate?" The Court's decision was based on the premise that, with time, a suspect may, in some unspecified way, ignore, forget, disregard, or view as insignificant a previous admission, embrace her right to remain silent and consult an attorney, and refuse to provide a second confession, despite having previously confessed. In the absence of empirical research on the attenuation effects of time between interrogations, we recommend that expert opinions should be offered cautiously, relying on the *totality of circumstances* that surrounded the interrogations.

Legal Procedures

Raising the Issue

The juvenile and criminal justice systems, which operate somewhat differently across jurisdictions, provide timetables for the provision of certain types of evidence and information. The prosecutor is expected to provide notice to the defense about the nature of the evidence against the defendant (e.g., provide defense counsel with a copy of the waiver and inculpatory statements it intends to introduce into evidence). Similarly, the defense must notify the prosecutor of evidence it intends to offer at trial. Typically, it is assumed that a defendant is capable of validly waiving his *Miranda* rights—unless the defense claims otherwise. If the defense chooses to challenge the validity of a *Miranda* waiver, the defense attorney must file a motion with the court asking for a pretrial suppression hearing. At the hearing, witnesses, including police interrogators and forensic mental health experts, may be called to testify. The prosecution bears the burden of proof to establish that *Miranda*

CASE LAW
Missouri v. Siebert (2004)

- The Court addressed the question of whether the rule from *Oregon v. Elstad* (1985), that a defendant who has made an un-Mirandized confession may later waive her Miranda rights to make a second confession (admissible in court), still applies when the initial confession is the result of an intentional decision by a police officer to withhold her Miranda warnings.

- The Court found that the post-Miranda confession is only admissible—even if the two-stage interview was unintentional—if the Miranda warning and accompanying break are sufficient to give the suspect the reasonable belief that she has the right not to speak with the police.

INFO

If the defense chooses to challenge the validity of a *Miranda* waiver, the defense attorney must file a motion with the court asking for a pretrial suppression hearing. It is at this hearing that the expert witness may be called to testify.

rights were waived in a legally valid manner. However, the standard of proof required varies across jurisdictions. For example, Colorado (*People v. Al-Yousif*, 2002; *People v. Trujillo*, 1993), Maine (*State v. Coombs*, 1998), Michigan (*People v. Daoud*, 2000), New York (*U.S. v. Miller*, 2005), Oklahoma (*Morris v. State*, 1988), and Tennessee (*State v. Kelly*, 1980) require a preponderance of the evidence, but Massachusetts requires a higher standard of proof—beyond a reasonable doubt (*Commonwealth v. Day*, 1983; *Commonwealth v. Jackson*, 2000). At the conclusion of the suppression hearing, the trial judge rules on the validity of the waiver. If the judge finds the waiver to have been validly executed, the confession can be introduced as evidence at trial. However, if the judge rules that the *Miranda* rights were not waived knowingly, intelligently, and voluntarily, the inculpatory statement is suppressed. If the statement is the only evidence implicating the defendant in the crime, charges generally are dropped.

If a judge rules that the waiver was valid and the confession admissible, most jurisdictions allow the defense to challenge the trustworthiness of the confession at trial (*Coyote v. United States*, 1967; *Jackson v. Denno*, 1964). Defendants, under the due process clause of the Fourteenth Amendment, can challenge evidence offered against them, including questioning the circumstances under which a confession was obtained. In *Lego v. Twomey* (1972), the U.S. Supreme Court held that to prove voluntariness, "the prosecution must prove at least by a preponderance of the evidence that the confession was voluntary. Of course, the States are free, pursuant to their own law, to adopt a higher standard." In Maine (*State v. Mikulewicz*, 1983), Minnesota (*State v. Anderson*, 1987) and New York (*People v. Huntley*, 1965), for instance, the state bears the burden of proving, beyond a reasonable doubt, that the waiver was made voluntarily.

In *Jackson v. Denno* (1964), the Court indicated, "a proper determination of voluntariness [must] be made prior to the admission of the confession to the jury. . . . " Only after the judge has ruled on the voluntariness of the waiver is the defendant granted the opportunity to challenge the confession before the jury. The jury does not decide on the admissibility of the statement but, rather, must consider how much weight, if any, to give to the confession based upon the circumstances in which it was obtained. As detailed in *Coyote v. United States*, "the jury should surely be told that if they find the defendant did not fully understand the meaning of the warning and advice given to him as stated in a confession, they may take that fact into consideration along with all the other facts and circumstances in determining the factual voluntariness of the statement" (see also *United States v. Inman*, 1965). In a New York case, *People v. Kogut* (2005), the court ruled that experts are permitted to testify about the methodology used to assess the voluntariness of a confession and about the research on the relationships between police interrogation practices and involuntary confessions; however, the court held that experts are not permitted to testify to the ultimate issue—whether a confession was voluntary or involuntary. Although *Kogut* was a state case, the prohibition against expert testimony on the ultimate issue on *Miranda* waivers is fairly consistent across jurisdictions.

Qualifications of the Expert

Experts must be declared as such by the judge hearing the case. *Jenkins v. United States* (1962) established that experts are those who (regardless of discipline) possess the background, skills, experience, training, or knowledge about the anticipated area of testimony; if admitted as an expert, the witness is permitted to offer opinions. The *Federal Rules of Evidence* (2001) incorporate these criteria. See chapter 7 for discussion about these sources of legal authority and their relevance to testifying about the validity of *Miranda* rights waivers.

INFO

In order to qualify the expert, the judge must determine that he possesses the necessary background, skills, experience, training, and knowledge.

Subject Matter of Expert Testimony

Experts can testify only about those topics or subjects that meet evidentiary standards (see chapter 7 for a detailed discussion of these standards and their impact on testimony). As Ewing (2003) indicated, expert testimony must be based, at least in part, on science. The federal government and many states use the criteria established by *Daubert v. Merrell Dow Pharmaceutical* (1993). Other states use, either exclusively or in combination with *Daubert*, the *Frye v. United States* (1923) standard of "general acceptance in the scientific community." Specifically, it is within each court's discretion to determine the admissibility and bounds of expert testimony (*People v. Cronin*, 1983). See chapter 7 for a discussion of the relevance of both the *Daubert* and *Frye* standards of admissibility to expert testimony on *Miranda* waiver validity. Regardless of the standard, experts should be aware that a judge may order a *Frye* or *Daubert* hearing if new methodology is used in an assessment or if unusual aspects or areas of testimony will be offered. At the hearing, the judge will rule on the admissibility of the proffered testimony.

Conclusions

This chapter provided an overview of significance of confessions in the legal process and the historical evolution of the rights to silence and legal counsel. *Miranda v. Arizona* was an integration of legal opinions that began with the exclusion of physically coerced testimony and included decisions that excluded psychologically coerced confessions, as well. Numerous court decisions reflect concerns about the likelihood that coerced or involuntary confessions increase the risk of innocent suspects admitting to crimes that they did not commit. Despite the initial application of *Miranda* rights to adults, the Court extended the rights to silence and counsel to juveniles as well. The *totality of circumstances* test for evaluating the validity of *Miranda* waivers was also applied to juvenile cases. The following chapters will discuss the significance of these legal decisions for structuring forensic mental health evaluations of defendants' capacities to waive their *Miranda* rights.

Forensic Mental Health Concepts | 2

This chapter reviews the forensic mental health interpretation of the criteria for a legally valid *Miranda* waiver. Specifically, it focuses on the ways in which the knowing and intelligent requirements of a valid rights waiver are translated into the forensic mental health concepts of understanding and appreciation, concepts that can be assessed during a forensic mental health evaluation. This chapter also describes the legal and conceptual difficulties of translating voluntariness into a forensic mental health concept. It also reviews courts' use of the *totality of circumstances* approach to evaluating the validity of a waiver.

For courts to evaluate whether *Miranda* rights waivers were made knowingly, intelligently, and voluntarily, these legal constructs must be translated into analogous forensic mental health concepts that can be assessed. Consequently, "knowing" is translated into "understanding," and "intelligent" is translated into "appreciation." "Voluntariness," is less directly translatable into a psychological construct, as it is much broader in scope, capturing both the characteristics of the interrogation and characteristics of the defendant.

To further define, "understanding" requires a basic comprehension of the meaning of the rights. If police delivered the rights in English, did the defendant understand English? If the police showed the defendant a written warning, could the defendant read? Did the defendant understand the vocabulary in the warning? Did the defendant understand the basic meaning of each of the rights in the warning?

"Appreciation" requires a greater level of comprehension. It is reflected in a defendant's abilities to have applied the *Miranda* rights to his own interrogation and to have grasped the potential consequences of waiving those rights. For example, even if a defendant "understands" what a lawyer is, did the defendant "appreciate" why he would want a lawyer and the potential consequences of not having one? Even if it the defendant "understands" that he has the right to remain silent, did he "appreciate" and grasp, during the interrogation, that a decision to remain silent could not be held against him by a judge?

"Voluntariness" is more difficult to translate into a single psychological construct; to be relevant to the legal decision a violation of "voluntariness" of the *Miranda* waiver must have been directly influenced by police coercion (*Culombe v. Connecticut*, 1961; *Colorado v. Connelly*, 1986; see chapter 1 for case law review). For the most part, the presence of physical or psychological coercion is a factual matter for which there may or may not be supporting evidence, such as a videotape of the interrogation. Nevertheless, evaluators can assess an individual's "susceptibility to police coercion." In other words, due to different attributes (e.g., age, IQ), personality characteristics (e.g., levels of suggestibility), and experiences (e.g., arrest history, educational history) of defendants, factors associated with the interrogation (e.g., length of the interrogation, police behaviors) may have been more or less likely to have resulted in a waiver and incriminating statement. Consequently, forensic mental health evaluators can assess the ways in which police behaviors and other characteristics of the interrogation could have influenced the defendant's susceptibility to coercion, *if* the alleged coercion actually occurred.

INFO

Some forms of police coercion are legally permissible, such as lying about evidence or the cooperation of witnesses, and cannot be taken into account when determining voluntariness as it relates to waiving Miranda rights.

It must be emphasized that during the course of an interrogation, police may mislead or lie to a suspect. As described by DeClue (2005), "When solid evidence is lacking, the interrogator relies entirely on deception and interpersonal dominance to gain a confession" (p. 19). DeClue cited examples of manipulative techniques used by police, including "reducing feelings of guilt; doing the right thing; showing empathy for the victim or the victim's family; maintaining the good will of the police; showing remorse to look good for the prosecutor, judge, or jury; or avoiding a harsh sentence such as a lengthy prison sentence or death" (p. 23). Interrogators may also misrepresent information about the nature of the evidence they have collected, statements provided to them by witnesses, and confessions offered of codefendants implicating the suspect. These procedures are generally considered to be legally permissible, and they would not represent a form of coercion affecting voluntariness (i.e., *Frazier v. Cupp*, 1969; *Haynes v. Washington*, 1963; *Schneckloth v. Bustamonte*, 1973).

2
chapter

Totality of Circumstances

In evaluating the validity of a *Miranda* waiver, courts use a *totality of circumstances* test to consider all of the factors surrounding an alleged *Miranda* violation (Grisso, 1998). No factors are mandatory for consideration, and no factor, by itself, would represent a reason for judges to rule, across cases, that *Miranda* rights were or were not legally waived.

This *totality of circumstances* approach dates back to the pre-*Miranda* period. Courts, recognizing coerced confessions as untrustworthy, used a voluntariness test of the admissibility of a confession, which was based on evaluation of the *totality of circumstances* that resulted in a given confession. This case-by-case voluntariness test allowed courts to consider the influence of a variety of factors, with early case law establishing consideration of background, experience, and conduct as appropriate (*Johnson v. Zerbst*, 1938).

Since the *Miranda* decision, courts have continued to use a *totality of circumstances* approach to evaluating the legal validity of a *Miranda* waiver and the admissibility of a confession. Case law (reviewed in chapter 1) has established a wide range of factors that may be considered when evaluating whether a waiver was provided knowingly, intelligently, and voluntarily. These factors are typically divided into two broad categories: 1) characteristics of the defendant at the time he provided the waiver, and 2) situational conditions of the interrogation (Grisso, 1998a).

Characteristics of the Defendant

Shortly after *Miranda*, *Coyote v. United States* (1967) provided a list of characteristics to be considered in determining defendants' capacities to have waived *Miranda* rights. Those characteristics related directly to the defendants' capacities included age, intelligence, education, amount of prior contact with police officers, conduct, and background. More recent case law has expanded the list of factors to be considered in the *totality of circumstances* approach (see Oberlander & Goldstein, 2001). Although no specific factors are required for consideration in the *totality of circumstances* test, courts usually do consider similar defendant-related factors, such as age, IQ, level of education, language ability, literacy, prior experience with the police, mental illness, and maturity (Frumkin, 2000; Goldstein et al., 2003; Grisso, 1981; Grisso, 1998b; Oberlander, 1998; Oberlander & Goldstein, 2001).

Situational Conditions of the Interrogation

In *Coyote v. United States*, the Court also specified characteristics of the interrogation context that should be considered when evaluating the *totality of circumstances* surrounding the confession, including police conduct and physical conditions. Again, no specific factors are required for consideration, but those characteristics of the interrogation typically considered by courts include whether the defendant was advised of the *Miranda* rights, number of times the *Miranda* warning was given, method of *Miranda* warning delivery (e.g., read aloud by an officer, read silently by the defendant, read aloud by the defendant, read and explained by an officer), methods police used to assess the defendant's comprehension of the warning prior to the waiver (e.g., no assessment, signed an acknowledgement that the warning was given, inquired whether the defendant waived each element of the warning, had the defendant waive each element of the warning in writing, asked the defendant to paraphrase each element of the warning), whether an interested adult was present during the interrogation, time elapsed between the warning's administration and interrogation, length of the interrogation, timing of the confession, the physical arrangements of the interrogation, and police strategies used during questioning (Grisso, 1981; Grisso, 1986; Oberlander, 1998; Oberlander & Goldstein, 2001; Oberlander, Goldstein, & Goldstein, 2003).

2
chapter

Linking Totality of Circumstances Factors to Capacity to Waive Miranda Rights

Miranda established that a legal waiver should be based on a "knowing, intelligent, and voluntary" waiver of rights. By extension, to establish an invalid waiver, an attorney must demonstrate that there were deficits in a defendant's abilities to have knowingly or intelligently waived his rights or that the confession was coerced and, therefore, involuntary. Consequently, when evaluating a defendant's capacity to have waived rights, one is only required to evaluate the degree to which the individual understood his rights, appreciated the significance of waiving those rights, and was susceptible to police coercion, if it occurred. There is no requirement to find a mental disease or defect or to link any factor to the deficits in understanding and appreciation or to susceptibility to coercive police behaviors.

Despite the lack of such a requirement, the trier of fact typically wants an explanation of why the defendant would

INFO

The following situational conditions of the interrogation are directly related to the defendant's capacity to waive Miranda rights:

- police conduct / strategies

- conditions of the interrogation (length, physical location, etc.)

- number of times the *Miranda* warning was given and how it was delivered (verbally, on paper, etc.)

INFO

You are only required to evaluate the defendant's comprehension and appreciation of his rights, and whether he was susceptible to coercion. You are not required to find mental defects or illness.

have had the identified understanding or appreciation deficits or susceptibility to police coercion. Consequently, it is critical to evaluate the *totality of circumstances* factors and determine the ways in which specific characteristics of the defendant and/or interrogation may have interfered with the defendant's understanding of rights, appreciation of rights, and/or susceptibility to coercive police behaviors.

Timing of the Evaluation Relative to the Interrogation

A suppression hearing can occur weeks, months, or even years after a confession was given during an interrogation. Courts are required to base their decisions about the admissibility of a confession on the legal validity of the *Miranda* waiver that occurred prior to the confession. Consequently, the trier of fact seeks information about a defendant's understanding, appreciation, and susceptibility to police coercion at the time of the interrogation—not at the time of the evaluation or hearing.

Between the time of interrogation and the time of the evaluation many factors can improve a defendant's understanding and appreciation of the *Miranda* rights and reduce his susceptibility to police coercion. For instance, the cognitive-developmental maturation associated with mere passage of time can improve an individual's understanding and appreciation and make him less susceptible to police pressure (Kalbeitzer, 2008). In addition, following the confession, arrest, and appointment of counsel, many attorneys will talk with their clients about the nature and content of the *Miranda* warning. Furthermore, the arrest and legal proceedings that follow a confession may teach a defendant, firsthand, in a very powerful, personally meaningful way, the consequences of waiving the rights to silence and counsel during interrogation. For other defendants, psychotropic medication may have been prescribed while incarcerated. The effects of medication may reduce or eliminate active psychotic symptoms that were present at the time the waiver was made, symptoms that may have interfered with *Miranda* comprehension.

Consequently, the evaluator must distinguish between comprehension of rights and potential susceptibility to police pressure at the time of interrogation and at the time of the evaluation. The evaluator may conclude that the defendant's understanding, appreciation, and susceptibility to police coercion at the time of evaluation are an overestimate of his understanding, appreciation, and susceptibility at the time he waived his *Miranda* rights and confessed. Chapter 6 presents specific recommendations for using evaluation data to make judgments about capacities at the time of interrogation.

Conclusions

When the forensic mental health professional evaluates a defendant's capacities to waive *Miranda* rights, he examines the defendant's understanding and appreciation of the *Miranda* warnings and characteristics of the defendant that may have made him susceptible to coercive police behaviors, if such behaviors occurred. Although a mental disease or defect is not required to explain deficits in understanding, appreciation, or susceptibility to coercive police behaviors, judges typically want explanations for such deficits or heightened susceptibility. Thus, the expert should examine the relevant *totality of circumstances* factors and whether any of these factors may be

INFO

Because a suppression hearing can occur long after the interrogation, by the time the defendant is evaluated he may have a better understanding and appreciation of Miranda rights due to consulting with an attorney or simply by going through the legal process. The evaluation must focus on the defendant's capacities at the time of the interrogation and not at the time of the evaluation or hearing.

linked to deficits in the defendant's capacities to have provided a knowing, intelligent, and voluntary waiver of rights. Furthermore, the expert must address the ways in which the defendant's *Miranda* comprehension and susceptibility to police pressure at the time of the evaluation reflect the defendant's capacities at the time that he provided the waiver in question.

Empirical Foundations and Limits | 3

This chapter reviews the empirical literature relevant to legal challenges to confessions based on questions about *Miranda* waivers. Specifically, this chapter presents information about the frequency of *Miranda* waivers, particularly among vulnerable populations, such as juveniles, adults with mental retardation, and adults with severe mental illness. It also reviews available data about the frequency with which *Miranda* waiver challenges are raised. A summary of the empirical literature is presented on the relationship between totality of circumstances factors and capacities required for a valid waiver of *Miranda*; particular emphasis is placed on the relationships between these totality of circumstances factors and the knowing and intelligent requirements of a valid rights waiver. In addition, we review the available assessment tools for evaluating these capacities in *Miranda* waiver evaluations; we present data about the psychometric properties of these instruments and their frequency of use and acceptability in the field, information that should be provided by the expert during an admissibility hearing.

How Often Do Suspects Waive Their Rights?

About 80% of suspects waive their rights (Leo, 1996; Cassell & Hayman, 1996), and over half of all suspects in the United States and England offer self-incriminating statements when questioned by police (Pearse & Gudjonsson, 1997). Adult suspects waive their rights at high rates, with estimates around that 80% mark (Kassin et al., 2007; Leo, 1996), but there are particular concerns about the rates at which juveniles, individuals with mental retardation, and those with mental illness seem to waive their rights. We discuss this in the next several sections.

Juvenile Suspects

Over three decades of research on juveniles' *Miranda* waivers has revealed that the vast majority of adolescent suspects waive their rights to silence and counsel. For instance, in two studies from the 1970s, over 90% of juveniles waived their *Miranda* rights (Ferguson & Douglas, 1970; Grisso & Pomicter, 1977). In the latter study, about 70% of the total number of juvenile felony arrests examined, involved police interrogation, and, in those cases, only 6.5% of youthful suspects refused to talk to police; the other suspects offered statements that contained some level of admission (approximately 85–90%) or denial (approximately 10%) of involvement in the offense (approximately 10%) (Grisso & Pomicter, 1977).

Despite the intervening 30 years, a twenty-first-century study of juvenile defendants produced similar rates of police interrogations, *Miranda* waivers, admissions, and denials during interrogations (Viljoen, Klaver, & Roesch, 2005). Seventy-five percent of youthful defendants reported having been questioned by police about the offense with which they were charged; only about 13% of those youth reported that they asserted the right to silence, and the remainder reported confessing (55%) or denying the offense (31%). Across the thirty-year time span, these rates of *Miranda* waivers occurred in spite of police reading most youth their rights and most youth remembering that they were read their rights (Grisso & Pomicter, 1977; Viljoen, Klaver, & Roesch, 2005).

Most research on the frequency of juveniles' *Miranda* waivers has focused on the waiver of the right to silence. However, it is clear that juveniles also waive the right to legal counsel in most cases. First, one can assume that if legal counsel were present, most youth would be instructed by their lawyers not to talk to police, and the aforementioned rates of confessions and denials suggest that lawyers were not present to offer guidance during interrogations. Second, empirical data supports the assumption that counsel is rarely present during juvenile interrogations. Of the 114 youth that had been questioned by police in one study, 10% reported having asked for a lawyer, but only one youth (less than 1%) reported having had an attorney present during questioning (Viljoen, Klaver, & Roesch, 2005).

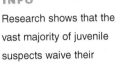

INFO

Research shows that the vast majority of juvenile suspects waive their Miranda rights.

Suspects with Mental Retardation

Little is known about the prevalence of *Miranda* waivers among individuals with mental retardation. The lack of data may be due, in part, to the fact that suspects are rarely identified as mentally retarded until after the interrogation process (Denkowski & Denkowski, 1985). Nonetheless, Rogers and Shuman (2005) offered a conservative estimate of over 400,000 suspects waiving their rights annually due to cognitive deficits. Notably, this number probably underestimates the frequency of waivers among mentally retarded suspects, given their disproportionately pronounced difficulties comprehending *Miranda* rights (e.g., Clare & Gudjonsson, 1991; Cloud, Shepherd, Barkoff, & Shur, 2002; Cooke & Phillip, 1998; Everington & Fulero, 1999; Fulero & Everington, 1995; O'Connell, Garmoe, & Goldstein, 2005), tendencies to produce socially desirable responses (Ellis & Luckasson, 1985), heightened suggestibility (e.g., Everington & Fulero, 1999) and tendencies to comply with authority figures (Shaw & Budd, 1982).

Suspects with Mental Illness

As with mental retardation, little data exist on the frequency of *Miranda* rights waivers by suspects with mental illness. Again, the identification of a mental illness usually does not occur until after the interrogation process. Nonetheless, a conservative estimate suggests that, annually, approximately 695,000 defendants suffer from a severe mental disorder when making waiver decisions (Rogers, Harrison, Hazelwood, & Sewell, 2007).

When defendants with severe mental disorders were asked to consider their cases retrospectively, one-quarter of defendants failed to produce a coherent, non-psychotic reason to exercise the right to silence; about 16% could not produce a coherent, nonpsychotic reason to exercise the right to counsel (Rogers, Harrison, Hazelwood, & Sewell, 2007). Although *Miranda* waiver frequency data for this population is largely unavailable, mentally ill suspects' difficulties understanding their rights (Cooper & Zapf, 2008) and appreciating the reasons for exercising their rights (Rogers, Harrison, Hazelwood, & Sewell, 2007) suggest that mentally ill suspects probably waive their rights more often than do non–mentally ill suspects.

Implications of Waiving Rights

Suspects who waive rights are at risk of providing incriminating information and, therefore, increasing their risks of conviction. In fact, many researchers and experts on *Miranda* waivers have reported that confessions are among the most powerful types of evidence at trial (e.g., Kassin, 1997; McCormick, 1972).

Beyond conviction, the waiving of rights can affect the severity of sentencing. For instance, youthful suspects who confess to police tend to be sentenced more harshly than do those youth who have not offered a confession (Ruback & Vardaman, 1997). Similarly, Leo (1996) found that adult suspects who provided confessions were more likely to receive punishment. These patterns clearly contradict any impressions suspects may have that cooperation with police questioning will result in leniency at sentencing.

Who is Referred for Miranda Assessment?

Most *Miranda* rights waivers are challenged based on questions about police delivery of the warnings (Grisso, 2003), challenges that have little to do with the characteristics of the suspects. Those cases involving challenges based on suspects' capacities to have waived rights suggest that the issue of *Miranda* rights

INFO

There is little evidence suggesting that cooperating with police leads to more lenient sentences. In fact, the opposite may be true.

waivers is most often raised when suspects have intellectual deficits or psychiatric diagnoses (Grisso, 2003).

How Often is the Issue Raised?

Little data are available to indicate the frequency with which attorneys question *Miranda* rights waivers, refer defendants for evaluations about capacities to have waived *Miranda* rights, or file motions to suppress confessions based on defendants' inabilities to meet the requirements of a knowing, intelligent, and voluntary waiver of rights. Of the data that are available in this area, most are related to juvenile cases and include information about all pretrial motions, not just motions to suppress confessions.

Such data have revealed that, in juvenile cases, motions to suppress under *Miranda* are rare (Juvenile Justice Center, 1995). Only 30% of the surveyed public defenders and appointed counsel who regularly represented juveniles reported regularly filing pretrial motions; confession suppression motions under *Miranda* are only one form of such motions. When explaining the reasons for not filing pretrial motions or aggressively trying cases, attorneys cited large caseloads, limited time, inadequate training, lack of professional support (e.g., specialized texts and computerized legal research, access to paralegals and bilingual staff or translators, adequate space for meeting with clients), and courthouse culture. According to these attorneys, many juvenile courts seem to emphasize the importance of facilitating the legal process, with many judges discouraging defense attorneys from embracing the adversarial role. The Juvenile Justice Center (1995) described how attorneys reported that in their jurisdictions they "do not file motions in order to maintain a 'friendly' atmosphere in the courthouse" and "only 'out-of-town' lawyers file motions. . . . " (p. 51).

Although still very limited, more data are available about the frequency with which *Miranda*-related motions to suppress confessions result in the loss of convictions. Across multiple cities and states, over numerous decades, it is clear that convictions are rarely lost as a result of suppression motions (see Cassell, 1996, for a thorough review of these data). First, motions to exclude confessions based on *Miranda* criteria succeed less than 1% of the time (Cassell, 1996). Second, in two separate studies of over 7000 and 3500 cases, respectively, only one conviction was lost in each study as a result of suppression motions to exclude confessions (Nardulli, 1983, 1987). Similarly, another study found that, at most, two of 619 cases, across two major cities, were dropped because of *Miranda* problems with confessions (Feeney, Dill, & Weir, 1983). Furthermore, on appeal, convictions are rarely reversed because of *Miranda*-related motions to suppress (Davies, 1982; Guy & Huckabee, 1988).

Thus, it appears that motions to suppress confessions under *Miranda* are rarely raised, rarely affect convictions, and rarely serve as the basis of successful appeals. Should defense attorneys be interested in challenging confessions under *Miranda* with greater frequency, data about suspects' understanding, appreciation, and assertion of rights could be helpful to their motions.

Relationship Between Totality of Circumstances Factors and Capacities to Waive Miranda Rights

As discussed in chapter 1, the *Miranda* (1966) decision required that suspects provide a waiver knowingly, intelligently, and voluntarily. When courts determine whether a waiver was valid (i.e., met these legal requirements), judges look to the totality of circumstances factors as legal indicants of these abilities (Grisso, 1981).

These totality of circumstances factors can focus on characteristics of the suspect and/or on characteristics of the interrogation. Suspect-related totality of circumstances factors include: (1) age, (2) intelligence, (3) education/literacy, (4) background, (5) mental illness/psychological symptoms, and (6) prior experience with police. Interrogation-related totality of circumstances factors include: (1) physical conditions of the interrogation and (2) police conduct. Notably, no single factor is indicative of adequate or inadequate. *Miranda* comprehension (Grisso, 1981).

In the sections that follow, we review the empirical research on the link between each of the totality of circumstances factors and *Miranda* understanding and appreciation (i.e., the analogous psychological constructs of the knowing and intelligent requirements of a valid rights waiver). We do not review the relationship between totality of circumstances factors and voluntariness because violations of the voluntariness requirement must be based on police coercion (*Colorado v. Connelly*, 1986)[1]. Therefore, voluntariness, generally, is not assessed directly by forensic evaluators during evaluations of defendants.

Suspect Characteristics

Age

When judges determine the admissibility of a confession, age and IQ seem to be critical factors considered among the totality of circumstances that could have interfered with defendants' capacities to have knowingly and intelligently waived rights. The critical role of age was seen in Grisso's (1981) review of juvenile (ages 9 to 19) appellate cases between 1948 and 1978, which raised the issue of juveniles' understanding of rights. In almost all cases involving defendants under age 13, judges decided that the defendants lacked sufficient understanding of their rights during interrogations. In cases involving 13- to 15-year-old defendants, judges' decisions were less consistent, and the cases produced the most dissenting opinions by judges. However, in three-quarters of cases involving 16- to 19-year-old defendants, judges determined that understanding of rights was sufficient. Although no recent research has systematically reviewed the role of age in courts' suppression decisions, experts in this area have observed that age continues to be a critical factor in judges' decision-making

1 Judges may consider the impact of defendant characteristics on voluntariness only if police exploited those characteristics to obtain a *Miranda* waiver.

about the admissibility of confessions (Oberlander, Goldstein, & Goldstein, 2003).

Consistent with judges' decision-making, age seems to be a primary factor in whether an individual chooses to invoke her rights. Overall, youth waive *Miranda* rights and offer confessions more often than do adults (e.g., Abramovitch, Peterson-Badali, & Rohan, 1995; Ferguson & Douglas, 1970; Grisso & Pomicter, 1977; Peterson-Badali, Abramovitch, Koegel, & Ruck, 1999; Viljoen, Klaver, & Roesch, 2005). Even among juveniles, there are significant age-related differences in the frequency of *Miranda* waivers, with younger adolescents at greater risk of waiving rights (e.g., Abramovitch, Higgins-Biss, & Biss, 1993; Abramovitch et al., 1995; Grisso & Pomicter, 1977; Viljoen, Klaver, & Roesch, 2005). In one study of juvenile defendants (ages 11 through 17), only about 8% of defendants under the age of 15 remained silent, with approximately 68% of defendants in this age group confessing during police questioning (Viljoen, Klaver, & Roesch, 2005). Regarding the right to counsel, no defendants under the age of 15 requested a lawyer (Viljoen, Klaver, & Roesch, 2005). Parallel statistics were not available for defendants ages 15 and over.

Although age seems to be associated with the frequency of *Miranda* waivers, a mere relationship between age and waiver frequency is not a sufficient basis for suppressing a confession under *Miranda*. Rather, a judge's determination that a *Miranda* waiver was invalid, in part due to age, requires a link between age and ability to provide a knowing, intelligent, and voluntary waiver of rights. To this end, age is one of the two variables (along with IQ) that have been most strongly and consistently linked to understanding of the *Miranda* rights warnings (e.g., Grisso, 1981; Goldstein, Morse, & Shapiro, 2003; Abromovitch et al., 1995), with juveniles demonstrating pronounced comprehension deficits, regardless of whether one uses a relative or absolute standard to determine adequate understanding and appreciation.

With respect to the relative standard, youth are less able to paraphrase and recognize the basic meaning of the *Miranda* warnings than are adults (e.g., Grisso, 1981; Abromovitch et al., 1995). They are also less able to define critical *Miranda* vocabulary than are adults and to appreciate the consequence of waiving rights (e.g., Grisso, 1981). Furthermore, younger adolescents demonstrate greater difficulties in these abilities than do older adolescents (e.g., Abromovitch et al., 1995; Colwell et al., 2005; Grisso, 1981; Goldstein et al., 2003; Viljoen & Roesch, 2005). For instance, in most studies, age was strongly related to *Miranda* understanding, up through about age 14 or 15, at which point a plateau was reached in the ability to understand the basic meaning of *Miranda* rights (e.g., Abramovitch et al., 1995; Goldstein et al., 2003; Grisso, 1981); in adulthood, age was unrelated to understanding of the warnings (Everington & Fulero, 1999; Grisso, 1981). However, the ability to define critical *Miranda* vocabulary words continued to improve with age, throughout adolescence and adulthood (Grisso, 1981). In terms of appreciation, juveniles under the age of 16 demonstrated significantly poorer grasps of the right to silence and counsel than did juveniles and adults, 20 years and over (Grisso, 1981).[2]

Although some judges are interested in how a defendant's understanding and appreciation compares with that of other defendants or community-based individuals (i.e., the relative standard), other judges are interested in the degree to which the defendant understands and appreciates the core, requisite information in the *Miranda* warnings (i.e., the absolute standard). With respect to the absolute standard, juveniles, as a group, cannot adequately paraphrase and recognize the critical information provided in the *Miranda* warnings, information that is central to providing an informed waiver of rights (e.g., Goldstein et al., 2003; Grisso, 1981). In addition, as a group, they cannot adequately define key words in the *Miranda* warnings (e.g., Goldstein, Condie, & Kalbeitzer, 2003; Grisso, 1981) nor are they able to adequately apply rights within an interrogation context and appreciate the consequences of waiving those rights (e.g., Goldstein et al., 2003; Grisso, 1981). These deficits are particularly pronounced for younger juveniles (e.g., Goldstein et al., 2003; Grisso, 1981). For example,

2 Juveniles' appreciation of the nature of interrogation did not differ significantly from that of adults.

in one study, approximately three-quarters of youth under the age of 13 and one-half of youth ages 13 to 15 inadequately understood their *Miranda* rights (as indicated by obtaining an inadequate rating on the paraphrasing of at least one of the four *Miranda* warnings) (Grisso, 1981). Youth also demonstrated great difficulty appreciating the significance of the warnings, with the majority of youth failing to adequately recognize that if a suspect refuses to talk to the police, the police must stop questioning. Similarly, over one-third of youth failed to adequately recognize that there would be no judicial penalty for asserting the right to silence, and more than half of the youth incorrectly believed that a judge could revoke this right (Grisso, 1981). Many also failed to appreciate the right to counsel, with more than one-quarter believing that a defense lawyer's role is to assist defendants who claim to be innocent, but not those who admit involvement in the offense (Grisso, 1981).

Notably, whether the suspect is guilty or innocent of an offense seems to moderate the relationship between age and assertion of the right to silence. In a vignette-based study, the decision to assert the right to silence was unrelated to guilt among younger youths (grades 6 and 8) and among young adults (university students); however, older youth (grades 10 and 13) were more likely to assert the right to silence if guilty than if innocent (Abramovitch et al., 1995). The researchers concluded that the older adolescents may have felt less need for legal protection when innocent. Guilt also seems to moderate the relationship between age and assertion of the right to counsel. Young adults said that they would get a lawyer more often when the suspect was guilty than when the suspect was innocent (Abramovitch et al., 1995), but school-aged participants were more likely to assert the right to counsel when innocent than when guilty. These differences in decision-making based on guilt may result from misunderstandings, in part tied to age, about the nature of rights, such as the commonly held belief that attorneys are only there to help the innocent (e.g., Grisso, 1981).

Although juveniles' understanding of rights is far worse than that of adults, even many adults are unable to fully understand the warnings (Clare & Gudjonsson, 1991; Grisso, 1981; Gudjonsson & Clare, 1994; Olley, Ogloff, & Jager, 1993; Shepherd, Mortimer, &

Mobasheri, 1995). For instance, in one study, more than half of the adult subjects were unable to provide an adequate definition of the word "right," describing it only as something one is allowed to do and failing to recognize the protectedness of a right (Grisso, 1981). Furthermore, approximately half of all adults incorrectly believed that a judge could revoke the right to silence, a misunderstanding that further demonstrates inadequate appreciation of the irrevocable nature of the right to silence. Why would a suspect choose to withstand the intense pressures from police during a prolonged interrogation if the suspect believes that she will be required to talk to the judge about the crime when she appears in court a few days later?

In sum, across 30 years of research, age has been strongly and consistently related to understanding and appreciation of *Miranda* rights. Specifically, age is related to the understanding of the basic meaning of the *Miranda* warnings, particularly in the younger adolescent years. Below the ages of 14 or 15, *Miranda* understanding improves dramatically with age, but improvements in understanding plateau between the ages of 14 and 16; however, there are notable individual differences within this older age range. In other words, if a defendant is under the age of 14, age alone will suggest a high probability that the defendant will not have understood her *Miranda* rights during interrogation. For defendants ages 14 through 16, many youth fail to demonstrate adequate understanding of rights, but information about other totality of circumstance factors must be examined, along with age, to make individually based predictions. Finally, although adults are presumed to understand and appreciate rights, many adults fail to grasp the significance of some central tenets of the *Miranda* rights; age, therefore, is not a good predictor of adults' *Miranda* comprehension, and other totality of circumstance factors are much more powerful in this age-group.

Developmental Factors

Cognitive, psychosocial, and neurological development may account, at least in part, for the age-related deficits in *Miranda* understanding and appreciation. Although cognitive, psychosocial, and neurological development occurs with age, there are individual differences in the speed of development and variability in the acquisition of specific, developmentally related skills, indicating that cognitive, psychosocial, and neurological maturity is not synonymous with age. Nonetheless, an understanding of cognitive, psychosocial, and neurological development can facilitate a broad understanding of some age-related *Miranda* deficits.

From a cognitive perspective, an informed *Miranda* waiver requires the suspect to have the abilities to understand the abstract concept of a right, interpret the complex implications of waiving rights, and weigh the costs and benefits of asserting and waiving the rights to silence and counsel. The development of such skills may be associated with age. For instance, thinking becomes more abstract and logical during the preteen and teenage years (Baird & Fugelsang, 2004). The ability to infer and weigh consequences associated with complex, imagined decisions is an advanced skill that requires this abstract thinking. Furthermore, there is empirical evidence that cognitive abilities, such as sustained attention (e.g., McKay, Halperin, Schwartz, & Sharma, 1994), verbal fluency (e.g., Levin et al., 1991), reasoning (e.g., Klaczynski, 2001), memory and learning (e.g., Levin et al., 1991; Ryan, 1990), and executive abilities (e.g., Davies & Rose, 1999) continue to develop through adolescence.

Regarding specific relationships between cognitive development and *Miranda* understanding and appreciation, age-related improvements in cognitive functioning (i.e., attention, verbal ability, general intellectual functioning, and executive functioning) partially explained age-related differences in *Miranda* understanding and appreciation in one study (Viljoen & Roesch, 2005). However, cognitive development did not entirely account for these differences, suggesting that other factors, such as psychosocial maturity, might explain some of the age-related differences in *Miranda* comprehension and reasoning.

Although psychosocial maturity has not been sufficiently operationalized as a psycho-legal construct (Cauffman & Steinberg, 2000; Salekin, Rogers, & Ustad, 2001; Salekin, Yff, Neumann, Leistico, & Zalot, 2002), research has identified developmentally related characteristics that affect the legal judgment and decision-making of adolescents (Colwell et al., 2005; Grisso et al., 2003; Scott, Reppucci, & Woolard, 1995; Steinberg & Cauffman, 1996). Cauffman and Steinberg (2000) proposed that such maturity of judgment, a primary component of psychosocial maturity, involves *Responsibility* (i.e., abilities to act independently, make decisions without the undue influence of others, and have a clear understanding of self); *Perspective* (i.e., abilities to weigh short- versus long-term consequences of decisions in a broad context and to see things from various point of view); and *Temperance* (i.e., ability to modulate impulsive thoughts and behaviors before acting). These psychosocial characteristics may relate differently to different types of legal judgments, depending on the demands of the legal situation and on other characteristics of the individual, such as intelligence (Cauffman & Steinberg, 2000; Colwell et al., 2005). Regarding *Miranda* waivers, a developed sense of autonomy, associated with Responsibility, may be required for a suspect to believe she has the right to assert her rights to silence and legal counsel, even when authority figures, such as police or parents, are pressuring her to talk with the police about the alleged offense. Similarly, a mature sense of Perspective might be needed for a youthful suspect to value the long-term benefits of remaining silent during a prolonged interrogation over the short-term benefit of confessing to end an unpleasant interrogation. And Temperance should help a youthful suspect inhibit her inclination to respond to police questions, so that she can consider her options and assert her rights to silence and counsel.

Research supports the role of psychosocial maturity in judgments about legal decisions, broadly (e.g., Grisso et al., 2003), and about *Miranda* understanding, appreciation, and decision-making, specifically (Colwell et al., 2005; Grisso et al., 2003). For instance, in one study, younger adolescents were less likely to recognize risks associated with legal decisions, less likely to recognize the long-term consequences of legal decisions, and more likely to comply with authority figures (Grisso et al., 2003). Specifically, 11 to 13 year olds reported fewer risks and long-range consequences associated with legal decisions than did older age groups.

Compared with older juveniles, youth ages 15 and younger were more likely to make decisions that seemed to comply with authority figures. In another study, psychosocial maturity was associated with understanding and appreciation of rights, with a particularly strong relationship between Responsibility and *Miranda* understanding and appreciation, even when controlling for age and IQ (Colwell et al., 2005). In other words, even after accounting for age and IQ, adolescents with higher scores on measures of self-reliance, internal control, and self-identity were better able to describe the meaning of the *Miranda* warnings, apply the warnings to interrogation scenarios, and appreciate the implications of waiving the rights to silence and counsel.

The cognitive and psychosocial maturity characteristics that explain some age-related differences in *Miranda* understanding, appreciation, and decision-making may be attributable to age-related variations in neurological development. A great deal of empirical evidence has indicated that brain structures and neurological mechanisms continue to mature throughout adolescence and into early adulthood. For instance, longitudinal neuroimaging research has revealed that the frontal lobes are the last part of the brain to reach maturity (Baird et al., 1999) and that frontal brain structures continue to develop (e.g., thinning of the gray matter, increases in white matter, neuronal myelination and pruning) throughout adolescence and are not fully formed until the twenties (Giedd et al., 1999; Gogtay et al., 2004; Sowell, Thompson, Holmes, Jernigan, & Toga, 1999). Researchers and scholars have concluded that the immaturity of adolescents' frontal lobes contributes to their psychosocial immaturity—their impulsivity, risk-taking tendencies, and vulnerability to peer pressure (e.g., Scott et al., 1995), characteristics that should decrease the ability to think through the meaning of rights and consequences of waiving rights, decrease the ability to withstand police pressure during interrogation, decrease the likelihood of asserting rights, and increase the likelihood of providing a confession.

In addition, the socio-emotional system of the brain, including the limbic and para-limbic regions (amygdala, nucleus accumbens, orbitofrontal cortex, medial prefrontal cortex, superior temporal sulcus) changes during puberty (Kambam & Thompson, 2009). Risky behavior may be more likely with increased accumbens activity, associated with the socio-emotional system during adolescence (Kambam & Thompson, 2009). Furthermore, because development of the cognitive controls that would regulate risk-taking behavior seems to lag behind the changes in the socio-emotional system, youth may be at particular risk for heightened risk-taking, reward-seeking, and sensation-seeking behaviors (Steinberg, 2008). Thus, during adolescence, youth may be particularly willing to risk the potential long-term negative consequences of waiving rights for the positive consequence of ending an unpleasant interrogation and potentially being released.

Furthermore, the increased sensitivity of the dopaminergic system that occurs during puberty may increase the reinforcing nature of specific situations, behaviors, or other stimuli (Steinberg, 2008). For instance, adolescents are highly susceptible to peer influence (Gardner & Steinberg, 2005; Steinberg & Monahan, 2007) and may find peer approval particularly rewarding. Theoretically, when police invoke the peer pressure of a fellow suspect to encourage a confession, the adolescent may be particularly at risk of waiving rights.

The American Medical Association amicus brief (American Medical Association et al., 2003) submitted in *Roper v. Simmons* (2005), the Supreme Court decision that excluded juveniles from capital punishment, noted that adolescents rely more on the amygdala (socio-emotional region) than on the prefrontal cortex (executive functioning region) and, as youth age, intensity of brain activity shifts from the amygdala to the frontal lobes. Although adolescents' diminished social and emotional abilities, decreased risk perception accuracy, and increased volatility were presented within the context of capital punishment, these same neurological factors may influence the understanding and appreciation of *Miranda* rights and decision-making about rights waivers.

Intelligence

Along with age, judges consider IQ a primary *totality of circumstances* factor when determining the admissibility of a confession.

For instance, in Grisso's (1981) review of juvenile appellate cases between 1948 and 1978, IQ scores were presented as evidence in about half of all cases that raised the issue of a juvenile defendant's understanding of rights. In nearly all of the cases in which judges determined that the defendants had lacked the requisite level of understanding for a valid waiver, the juvenile defendants had IQ scores below 75. Although there do not appear to be data on the role of IQ in judges' considerations of the validity of adults' Miranda waivers, research suggests that adults with mental retardation may frequently confess to police during interrogations without fully understanding their rights (see Everington & Fulero, 1999, and Fulero & Everington, 2004).

Across studies, along with age, IQ has been the totality of circumstances factor most closely associated with *Miranda* understanding and appreciation. Often, IQ has been an even stronger predictor of rights comprehension than has age. For instance, among juvenile justice youth, over a 30-year period, IQ has been strongly associated with the abilities to paraphrase rights and recognize the meaning of rights (Colwell et al., 2005; Goldstein et al., 2003; Grisso, 1981; Viljoen & Roesch, 2005). Although IQ has also been associated with the generalized ability to appreciate the consequences of waiving rights, it seems to be more strongly related to the appreciation of the right to silence and right to counsel than to the appreciation of the nature of interrogation (Colwell et al., 2005; Grisso, 1981). Although many studies have looked at Full Scale IQ scores, verbal intelligence (i.e., VIQ) seems to be particularly strongly associated with *Miranda* understanding and appreciation (Colwell et al., 2005; Viljoen & Roesch, 2005).

Notably, the importance of IQ to *Miranda* understanding and appreciation seems to vary by age. Grisso's (1981) research suggested that, among juvenile justice youth, IQ may be most influential in the 14- to 16-year-old age range. Below that age, most youth were unable to understand rights, regardless of IQ, and, above that age, juveniles' understanding more closely paralleled that of adults (Grisso, 1981). Despite this finding, Viljoen and Roesch (2005) more recently found that, among their sample of 11- to 17-year-old defendants, younger juveniles' understanding was far more dependant on intelligence than was the understanding of older juveniles. This discrepancy, along with the consistent finding that, among juvenile justice youth, intelligence was an important predictor of understanding and appreciation across age groups (Colwell et al., 2005; Goldstein et al., 2003; Grisso, 1981; Viljoen & Roesch, 2005;), suggests that the potential impact of both age and IQ on *Miranda* understanding and appreciation should be examined when evaluating a defendant's capacity to have waived rights during interrogation.

Among adult offenders and nonoffenders, *Miranda* understanding was primarily related to differences in IQ scores, even while controlling for age, gender, race, and socioeconomic status (SES) (Grisso, 1981). The role of IQ in *Miranda* comprehension is particularly notable in the lowest IQ ranges. Many studies have found that cognitively impaired individuals often fail to comprehend the *Miranda* warnings, particularly relative to nonimpaired populations (e g , Clare & Gudjonsson, 1991; Cloud, Shepherd, Barkoff, & Shur, 2002; Cooke & Phillip, 1998; Everington & Fulero, 1999; Fulero & Everington, 1995; O'Connell, Garmoe, & Goldstein, 2005). In fact, understanding among adults with mental retardation was lower than among the juveniles in Grisso's (1981) study (Fulero & Everington, 1995). For instance, 90% of adults with mental retardation in a workshop setting, and 67% of adults with mental retardation on probation, demonstrated an inadequate understanding of rights. In fact, of the adults on probation, more than half of those with mental retardation demonstrated inadequate understanding of the right to silence and intended use of self-incriminating information in court (compared with 3% and 10% of nonretarded adult probationers, respectively). A total of 39% of probation adults with mental retardation demonstrated inadequate understanding of the right to counsel, and 17% demonstrated inadequate understanding of the right to counsel for indigent defendants (versus 8% and 7% for nonretarded adult probationers, respectively).

Another study of adults with mild mental retardation produced even higher rates of deficits in *Miranda* comprehension (O'Connell et al., 2005). Some 50% of participants demonstrated inadequate understanding of all five *Miranda* rights when asked to paraphrase their meaning. Even when asked to recognize the meaning of rights using a forced choice format, only 2% of participants scored better than chance. Notably, this level of deficit far exceeds Grisso's (1998) findings that less than 1% of adults in the general population demonstrated inadequate understanding when asked to paraphrase four warnings, and approximately 75% of adults in the general population scored above chance when asked to recognize the meaning of rights (O'Connell et al., 2005).

Although few studies have focused on the role of IQ in the *Miranda* comprehension of mentally ill defendants, the extant research in this area also suggests that IQ is a critical predictor of the legal capacities required for a valid rights waiver. For adult psychotic defendants, IQ was the strongest predictor of the understanding of interrogation rights (Viljoen, Roesch, & Zapf, 2002). Thus, it seems clear that, across the populations identified as most at-risk for providing an invalid *Miranda* waiver, IQ is a critical factor—possibly the *most* critical—among the *totality of circumstances* factors for providing a knowing and intelligent waiver of rights.

Education and Literacy

HISTORY OF SPECIAL EDUCATION

Grisso (1981) found that, in a few of the juvenile appellate cases in which *Miranda* understanding was viewed as inadequate, judges explicitly cited placement in a classroom for students with mental retardation as evidence of very low intelligence and poor understanding. To our knowledge, there are only two studies that have empirically examined the relationship between special education history and *Miranda* comprehension.

The first study found that the *Miranda* comprehension of delinquent males who reported having participated in special education programs was significantly lower than the comprehension of delinquent males who said that they had never participated in special education programming (Goldstein et al., 2003). However, participation was unrelated to self-reported likelihood of offering false confessions in a variety of police interrogation scenarios.

In the second study, an extension of the first, special education was not related to *Miranda* understanding or appreciation (Riggs Romaine, Zelle, Wolbransky, Zelechoski, & Goldstein, 2008). Given the wide variety of reasons for placement in special education (e.g., low IQ, learning disabilities, mental health issues, behavioral problems), there may be great variability in the relationship between special education and *Miranda* comprehension across samples (Riggs Romaine et al., 2008). Individual academic skills that are relevant to *Miranda* comprehension might be a better indicator of understanding and appreciation of rights.

READING AND LISTENING COMPREHENSION

In his juvenile appellate review, Grisso (1981) found that, in the few cases in which reading abilities were cited, judges determined that youth with reading comprehension scores at a fifth grade level or higher had adequate *Miranda* understanding. In these cases, reading comprehension seems to have been used as an indicator of general intellectual capacity. However, based on more general research on reading abilities, Greenfield and colleagues (2001) concluded that if the reading level of a *Miranda* warning exceeds the individual's reading level by at least two grades, the validity of the *Miranda* waiver may be questionable. Given the wide variability in the reading levels of *Miranda* warnings (e.g., Rogers, Harrison, Shuman, Sewell, & Hazelwood, 2007; Rogers, Hazelwood, Sewell, Shuman, & Blackwood, 2008), many suspects who read at the fifth-grade level may not adequately comprehend their rights.

An empirical review of the relationship between specific academic achievement skills and *Miranda* comprehension revealed that, in addition to age and IQ, academic achievement was the strongest predictor of *Miranda* comprehension (Zelle, Riggs Romaine, Serico, Wolbransky, Osman, Taormina, Wrazien, & Goldstein, 2008). Specifically, even when controlling for age and verbal IQ scores, composite measures of reading and language abilities were each significantly associated with the ability to explain the meaning of rights, with reading comprehension and composite language scores also associated with appreciation of rights. Notably, delinquent youth with reading abilities (basic reading and reading comprehension) below the fourth grade level demonstrated a significantly poorer understanding of rights than did peers with reading abilities at the fifth-grade level or higher.

Thus, it appears that academic achievement is an important factor to assess when evaluating *Miranda* comprehension. Notably, highest academic grade completed should not be used as a proxy for education level, as many post-schooling factors can affect educational abilities (Greenfield et al., 2001). Instead, specific academic abilities (e.g., reading comprehension, listening comprehension) should be directly examined as close as possible to the time of the *Miranda* waiver in question.

Background

GENDER

Nearly all of the studies that have examined gender differences in *Miranda* comprehension have found no differences between males' and females' understanding and/or appreciation of rights, regardless of whether the study examined juvenile justice youth (Goldstein et al., 2003; Grisso, 1981), school-based samples of youth (Abramovitch et al., 1995[3]), adult offenders and nonoffenders (Grisso, 1981), or adult probationers with or without mental retardation (Everington & Fulero, 1999).

However, one study did find that female juvenile defendants demonstrated poorer appreciation of the right to silence than did adolescent male defendants (Viljoen & Roesch, 2005). The researchers concluded that the gender difference may be attributable to the fact that female youth in the study reported having spent less time with their attorneys, a factor that was significantly related to understanding and appreciation of *Miranda* rights.

---

[3] Although Abramovitch, Peterson-Badali, and Rohan (1995) found no gender differences in the understanding of the rights to silence and counsel among students in grades 6 through 13, they did find a significant three-way interaction between Guilt, Evidence, and Gender on assertion of rights in their vignette-based study. Youth of both genders were more likely to assert their right to silence when the character in the vignette was guilty than when the character was innocent. However, the males were more likely to do so when told that the evidence against them was strong, and the females were more likely to assert their right to silence when told that the evidence against them was weak. Despite this significant interaction, post-hoc analyses revealed no significant gender differences in pairwise comparisons.

RACE/ETHNICITY

Most studies that have examined racial and ethnic differences in *Miranda* understanding and appreciation have produced results suggesting that there is no simple relationship between these variables. When controlling for age and IQ, studies have typically found no generalized racial or ethnic differences in *Miranda* understanding or appreciation among a variety of populations, including juvenile offenders (Goldstein et al., 2003; Grisso, 1981), adult offenders and nonoffenders (Grisso, 1981), and adult probationers with and without mental retardation (Everington & Fulero, 1999).

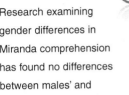

INFO

Research examining gender differences in Miranda comprehension has found no differences between males' and females' understanding and/ or appreciation of rights.

Although no simple relationships have been found between race or ethnicity and *Miranda* comprehension, some studies have found more complex ones. For instance, in one study, among juveniles with low IQ scores (i.e., below 80), African American juveniles exhibited poorer understanding and appreciation of rights than did White youth (Grisso, 1981); this racial difference seemed to be confined primarily to juveniles with a combination of below-average intelligence and lower or lower-middle SES backgrounds. Although another study produced no ethnic differences across the range of racial and ethnic groups, African American youth demonstrated better *Miranda* comprehension than did Latino youth (Goldstein et al., 2003).

Furthermore, these same two studies found that ethnicity moderated the relationship between arrest history and *Miranda* comprehension. In the first study, White juvenile offenders with three or more felony charges demonstrated better *Miranda* comprehension than did those offenders with few or no felony charges; conversely, African American youth with three or more felony referrals demonstrated poorer comprehension (Grisso, 1981). Similarly, in the second study, although the relationship between number of previous arrests and *Miranda* comprehension varied by ethnicity, the pattern was uninterpretable (Goldstein et al., 2003). Nonetheless, the more times Latino juvenile offenders reported

3 chapter

that they had been detained and given the *Miranda* warning (up to five detainments), the worse their *Miranda* comprehension; this pattern was not found with other ethnic groups.

In sum, it appears that relationships between race or ethnicity and *Miranda* understanding and appreciation are probably not simple or direct. They seem to vary with the culture of the neighborhood, cultural composition of the police forces with which the youth have experience, or recent treatment of particular racial or ethnic groups in the relevant geographic area.

SES

Although race and SES are closely related in the United States (e.g., Bishaw & Iceland, 2003; Harrison & Bennett, 1995), some studies have separately evaluated the relationship between SES and *Miranda* comprehension, and others studies have even attempted to sort out this relationship, independent of race.

One study found that juvenile defendants were less likely to assert the rights to silence and counsel if they were from low SES backgrounds (Viljoen, Klaver, & Roesch, 2005). The researchers explained that this finding might be due to the fact that children from low SES backgrounds are less likely to believe that they are entitled to rights and less likely to have opportunities to practice asserting rights (Melton, 2008). Consistent with this finding, juvenile defendants from low SES backgrounds demonstrated poorer understanding and appreciation of *Miranda* rights, even after controlling for cognitive abilities, psychological symptoms, and attorney contact (Viljoen & Roesch, 2005).

Despite these findings, earlier research did not find a relationship between SES and *Miranda* comprehension among juvenile offenders, adult offenders, or adult nonoffenders, when controlling for age, IQ, gender, and race (Grisso, 1981). Thus, the role of SES, as a *totality of circumstances* factor in the evaluation of *Miranda* understanding and appreciation, should be considered with extreme caution.

Mental Illness and Psychological Symptoms

A fundamental assumption of mental health law is that mental disorder puts individuals at risk for legal impairment (see Winick, 1996), and rates of police contact with mentally ill individuals are disproportionately high (e.g., Bonovitz & Bonovitz, 1981; Pogrebin & Poole, 1987; Schellenberg, Wasylenki, Webster, & Goering, 1992; Teplin, 1983). Indeed, one study found that individuals showing symptoms of mental illness are 67 times more likely to be arrested than are those without symptoms (Teplin, 2000).

When determining a defendant's capacity to have waived rights, *Miranda* experts recommend considering the presence of mental illness or a psychotic condition at the time of interrogation (Frumkin, 2000; Grisso, 2003). Although mental illness is not a requirement for determining that a defendant did not have the capacities to waive his rights during interrogation—it is just one of the many totality of circumstances factors to consider—U.S. courts have indicated concerns about the waiver capacities of mentally ill suspects (Viljoen & Roesch, 2005).[4]

Among adult inpatients, the types of *Miranda*-related errors in understanding and appreciation are fairly similar to those of youth and individuals with cognitive deficits. For instance, approximately 60% of patients failed to understand at least one *Miranda* right (Cooper & Zapf, 2008). Furthermore, approximately half of the psychiatric inpatients in the aforementioned study reported believing that a judge can revoke a defendant's right to silence when the defendant appears in courts (Cooper & Zapf, 2008). When asked why a defendant would have to talk to a judge about what he did wrong, common answers were "You have to prove you are innocent"; "If you don't talk you will get jail time"; and "You have to talk if you are under oath" (Cooper & Zapf, 2008, p. 401). Notably, these rates of errors may be an underestimate, as psychiatric patients who were

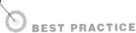

BEST PRACTICE
When determining a defendant's capacity to have waived rights, be sure to consider the presence of mental illness or a psychotic condition at the time of interrogation.

---

4 In a number of other countries (e.g., England, Wales, Australia), the concerns about the vulnerability of mentally ill suspects are so strong that an appropriate adult or independent third party must be present when police interview a mentally disordered suspect (e.g., Gudjonsson, 1993, 1995; Pearse, 1995; Robertson, Pearson, & Gibb, 1996).

unable to provide informed consent were excluded from the study, and patients who had had mental health symptoms in the previous two weeks, but not necessarily at the time of *Miranda* testing, were classified as disordered.

PSYCHOTIC SYMPTOMS

Most of the court decisions and much of the research on mental illness and capacity to waive rights has focused on the presence of psychotic symptoms. Overall, most studies have found that criminal justice–involved adults with psychotic disorders demonstrate poorer comprehension of rights than do nonpsychotic individuals from similar comparison groups. More specifically, inmates with a history of psychotic disorders showed poorer understanding of rights than did nondisordered inmates, although appreciation did not differ between groups (Olley, 1998). Similarly, among adult inpatients, even when accounting for IQ, those individuals with a diagnosis of psychosis scored lower than those patients without a psychotic diagnosis on all measures of *Miranda* understanding and appreciation (Cooper & Zapf, 2008). These adult inpatients appeared more impaired on measures of understanding and appreciation of rights than either adult offenders or adults from the community; they appeared, generally, to score similarly to or lower than juvenile offenders and only slightly better than mentally retarded adults in other studies (Cooper & Zapf, 2008).

Another study, which also controlled for IQ, revealed that adult defendants with psychotic disorders displayed poorer recognition of the meaning of rights than did nonpsychotic defendants, although abilities to paraphrase rights and define *Miranda*-related vocabulary did not differ between groups (Viljoen, Roesch, & Zapf, 2002). Such skills may depend on language abilities that are less susceptible to deterioration as a result of mental disorders and aging (Gold & Harvey, 1993; Heinrichs & Zakzanis, 1998; Horn & Hofer, 1992; Lezak, 1983). Recognition, in contrast, may depend more on attention and working memory, skills that may be more susceptible to mental state (Viljoen, Roesch, & Zapf, 2002). Examining *Miranda* comprehension within the spectrum of severe mental illness, defendants with schizophrenia demonstrated poorer understanding of rights than did defendants with other psychotic disorders (Viljoen, Roesch, & Zapf, 2002).

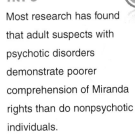

Although most research has revealed a relationship between psychosis and *Miranda*-impairment, one study failed to detect such a relationship (Rogers, Harrison, Hazelwood, & Sewell, 2007). Among pretrial defendants on competency to stand trial units, this study found no effect of psychosis on *Miranda* understanding, and the authors concluded that cognitive variables outperformed diagnostic variables as predictors of *Miranda* comprehension. This study did, however, find extensive impairment in understanding of all but the simplest *Miranda* warnings among mentally disordered defendants, in general; it also found that Global Assessment of Functioning (GAF) scores were significantly associated with *Miranda* comprehension.

DEPRESSION

Given that clinical depression is associated with cognitive processing deficits (see Mineka, Rafaeli, & Yovel, 2003), researchers and legal scholars have theorized that depressed individuals may be less inclined to assert rights, less resistant to challenge interrogators, and less able to accurately judge how well they are fulfilling their goals in an interrogation (Follette, Davis, & Leo, 2007). Furthermore, the depression-related distortions of self-worth (King, Naylor, Segal, Evans, & Shain, 1993), inaccurate estimates of performance in a variety of social situations (Gable & Shean, 2000), and hopelessness about the future (MacLeod, Rose, & Williams, 1993), may reduce depressed suspects' motivation to consider the meaning of rights, to appreciate the consequences of waiving rights, and to stand up to police by asserting rights.

Despite the strong theoretical relationships between depressive symptoms and *Miranda* capacities, we are aware of only two studies that have empirically examined this relationship, one with juvenile offenders (Olubadewo, 2009) and the other with adult defendants (Viljoen & Roesch, 2005). Neither study found a significant association between depression and *Miranda* understanding or appreciation.

ANXIETY

As with depression, there is a strong theoretical relationship between clinical anxiety and *Miranda*-related capacities. It has been proposed that individuals with anxiety would find the stress of an interrogation so aversive that they would seek a quick end to the proceedings (e.g., provide a confession), even if that meant future negative consequences (Follette, Davis, & Leo, 2007). Furthermore, anxiety interferes with effective cognitive processing (e.g., Covington & Omelich, 1987), and stressful situations heighten suggestibility (e.g., Gudjonsson & Singh, 1984). Thus, *Miranda* understanding, appreciation, and decision-making might be compromised by clinical anxiety, which, theoretically, would be exacerbated by the unique stress of an interrogation.

We are aware of only two studies that have empirically examined the relationships between clinical anxiety and *Miranda* capacities (Olubadewo, 2009; Viljoen and Roesch, 2005), and neither found significant associations. Notably, over half of the adolescent defendants in one study reported that they felt worried at the time of police questioning (Viljoen, Klaver, & Roesch, 2005).

ATTENTION DEFICIT HYPERACTIVITY DISORDER (ADHD)

The deficits in attention allocation, impulse control, and self-monitoring associated with ADHD (Redding, 2006) could be linked to deficits in *Miranda* capacities. In theory, attention deficits should interfere with a suspect's abilities to focus on and process the reading of rights, interpret the meaning of rights, and consider the implications of waiving those rights; it could also limit a suspect's ability to detect the antagonistic nature of police questioning. Furthermore, the impulsivity and hyperactivity associated with ADHD should, theoretically, interfere with a suspect's capacity to inhibit verbal responses to police questions and to think through the implications of their answers before responding. In addition, the self-monitoring deficits associated with ADHD could interfere with suspects' abilities to present themselves in socially desirable, nonincriminating ways.

To our knowledge, only one study has examined the relationship between ADHD symptoms and *Miranda* capacities. Research with adolescent defendants, ages 11 to 17, revealed that youth with attention deficits, hyperactivity, and psychomotor agitation were more likely to waive the right to counsel than were those youth without these symptoms (Viljoen, Klaver, & Roesch, 2005). In a study with adult defendants, attention was significantly related to *Miranda* understanding and appreciation (Viljoen & Roesch, 2005).

SUBSTANCE USE

Approximately 40% of delinquent youth in a 1970s study reported that they were under the influence of alcohol or drugs at the time that they spoke with police and were arrested (Ferguson & Douglas, 1970). Similarly, in a 2005 study, many adolescent defendants reported having been drunk or high at the time of police questioning (Viljoen, Klaver, & Roesch, 2005). Within a group of adult suspects, confession rates were higher among those suspects who reported having consumed illicit drugs in the 24 hours prior to interrogation (Pearse, Gudjonsson, Clare, & Rutter, 1998).

To our knowledge, only one study has examined the relationship between substance use and *Miranda* comprehension, finding that juvenile offenders' self-reports of alcohol and drug use were significantly associated with deficits in *Miranda* understanding (Olubadewo, 2009). In addition, many studies have examined the relationships between intoxication and skills that should, theoretically, be pertinent to adequate understanding and appreciation of rights. For instance, intoxication reduces inhibition, attention, reasoning, and self-monitoring, and it increases impulsivity and risk-taking (e.g., Fromme, Katz, & D'Amico, 1997; Hull & Young, 1983); such executive functioning deficits should, theoretically, interfere with a suspect's abilities to understand *Miranda* rights, appreciate the significance of waiving rights, and make informed decisions during police interrogations.

Beyond the effects of intoxication, substance-abusing suspects may be particularly at risk for invalid *Miranda* waivers. For example, substance-abusing patients tend to be impulsive, valuing a short-term, smaller reward over a delayed, larger reward (see Madden, Bickel, & Jacobs, 1999); in experimental settings, heroin addicts' discounting of delayed rewards was almost identical to that of 12-year-olds. Such tendencies could result in a suspect confessing to obtain the short-term reward of ending an unpleasant interrogation at the expense of providing self-incriminating information for use at a future hearing or trial. Although substance abuse and *Miranda* waiver capacities are theoretically related, however, apparently no research has evaluated the direct relationship between them.

PERSONALITY DISORDERS AND PERSONALITY CHARACTERISTICS

Cluster B personality disorders (antisocial, borderline, histrionic, and narcissistic personality disorders) are characterized by some degree of dramatic, emotional, or erratic behavior (DSM-IV-TR, 2000). There is reason to believe that stressful situations, like police interrogations, increase the probability that people with some Cluster B personality disorders will fail to successfully regulate thoughts, emotions, and behaviors (Follette, Davis, & Leo, 2007).

Although research on the relationship between personality disorders and *Miranda* comprehension has been virtually nonexistent, some personality characteristics have been found to correlate significantly with the reasons offenders give for having confessed to police. Among both juvenile offenders and adult inmates, anxiety proneness (neuroticism) and compliance correlated significantly with an internal need to confess and, to a lesser extent, with perceptions of external police pressure during interrogation (Gudjonsson & Sigurdsson, 1999).

Prior Experience with Police

Generally, courts seem to consider a history of arrest as an indicator of sufficient *Miranda* understanding, as judges may believe that such a history has provided exposure to the *Miranda* warnings and direct opportunities to learn the meaning of the warnings and consequences of waiving *Miranda* rights (Grisso, 1981).

Despite this fairly consistent legal judgment, research has repeatedly suggested that more extensive histories of arrest do not translate directly into better *Miranda* comprehension, regardless of whether this relationship is examined with juveniles (Goldstein et al., 2003; Grisso, 1981), adults (Grisso, 1981), or adults with mental illness (Cooper & Zapf, 2008; Viljoen & Roesch, 2005). Although one study did find a difference in *Miranda* understanding between probation and community samples of adults with mental retardation, the study did not control for IQ (Fulero & Everington, 1995).

Although *Miranda* comprehension, generally, does not differ based on arrest history, a few studies have found some differences in specific aspects of understanding and appreciation. For instance, although the number of prior felony arrests was not associated with better appreciation among juveniles when considered broadly, it was associated with somewhat better appreciation of the nature of the attorney-client relationship and the significance of the right to silence when IQ was taken into account. Among juvenile justice youth, juveniles with extensive arrest histories (i.e., three or more felony arrests) better appreciated the right to counsel than did youth with only one or two felony arrests (Grisso, 1981). Although offending and nonoffending adults did not differ in *Miranda* understanding, among adult offenders, the number of prior felony arrests was significantly related to the ability to paraphrase rights, but not to the abilities to recognize the meaning of rights or define *Miranda* vocabulary (Grisso, 1981). In one study, adult offenders better appreciated the right to silence than did adult nonoffenders, although there seemed to have been no difference in appreciation of this right between adults with one previous arrest and those with more extensive arrest histories (Grisso, 1981). However, in another study of adult defendants, the number of previous arrests was associated with appreciation of the right to counsel (Viljoen & Roesch, 2005).

Although repeated exposure to the *Miranda* warnings at the time of police questioning might result in increased familiarity with the warnings, it does not appear to result in increased understanding or appreciation. First, interrogations are stressful, and anxiety

INFO

Although repeated exposure to the *Miranda* warnings at the time of police questioning might result in increased familiarity with the warnings, it does not appear to result in increased understanding or appreciation.

interferes with the learning of verbal material (Torren et al., 2000). Second, the concept of a "right" is fairly abstract, and individuals may require a certain level of cognitive development, psychosocial development, and general cognitive functioning (e.g., reading comprehension, listening comprehension) to be able to understand and appreciate rights, regardless of their frequency of exposure. Third, experiences with interrogation and arrest may be inconsistent with the significance of *Miranda* rights (e.g., Moston, Stephenson, & Williamson, 1992), resulting in greater difficulty understanding them and appreciating their significance; for instance, confessions to minor offenses may actually result in a quick end to an interrogation and fairly rapid processing and release, particularly for young and/or first-time offenders.

In contrast to the lack of relationship between mere exposure to and comprehension of the *Miranda* warnings, history of contact with attorneys does appear to be strongly associated with both understanding and appreciation. Regardless of whether this history is measured as a yes/no variable or as the amount of time spent with an attorney, the relationship is strong. Notably, this relationship held even for younger youth and youth with low IQ scores (Viljoen & Roesch, 2005). Perhaps attorneys directly or indirectly explain rights to their clients (e.g., "Don't talk to anyone about the crime, no matter who it is or what they say to you"), warn them about the implications of waiving rights (e.g., "If you tell anyone in jail about what you did, she'll tell the judge and you'll get in a lot of trouble when you go to court"), and

INFO

Unlike repeated exposure to Miranda rights during police questioning, history of contact with attorneys appears to be strongly associated with both understanding and appreciation of rights.

develop a first-hand appreciation of the role of the attorney (e.g., defendants see their attorneys advocating for them, regardless of their guilt). In other words, clients may be directly exposed to the meaning and significance of *Miranda* rights through their contacts with attorneys, rather than merely exposed to the words of the warning, as they are during police questioning.

Situational Conditions of the Interrogation

Characteristics of the interrogation can interfere with the ability to understand and appreciate rights, and they may also influence decisions about whether to assert or waive rights. These potential influences will be described in this section.

Physical Condition

LENGTH OF INTERROGATION AND SLEEP LOSS

In theory, the prolonged stress created by a lengthy interrogation could interfere with a suspect's ability to think clearly about the meaning of rights, appreciate the significance of waiving rights, and make a logical and informed decision about whether to waive rights. Furthermore, the confusion generated by mixed messages from police during questioning might further interfere with understanding, appreciation, and informed decision-making. Police statements that an interrogation will end if the suspect answers police questions may be particularly persuasive after many hours of an unpleasant interrogation.

In addition to the stress that can be generated by lengthy interrogations, sleep deprivation may also occur. Sleep loss has been associated with a number of cognitive skills that should be critical to the semantic interpretation of *Miranda* rights, consideration of the consequences of waiving rights, and decision-making processes needed to make an informed waiver of rights. For instance, sleep loss decreases thinking and processing speeds (Dinges & Kribbes, 1991; McCarthy & Waters, 1997), reduces concentration (Williams, Lubin, & Goodnow, 1959), negatively impacts selective attention (Hockey, 1970; Norton, 1970), interferes with the ability to ignore irrelevant information (Blagrove,

Alexander, & Horne, 1995), decreases verbal fluency and flexibility (Horne, 1988; Randazzo, Muehlbach, Schweitzer, & Walsh, 1998; Wimmer, Hoffmann, Bonato, & Moffitt, 1992), and reduces frontal lobe functioning in tasks of word fluency, sentence completion, and semantic flexibility (Harrison & Horne, 1996). It also increases impulsivity in complex decision-making (Harrison & Horne, 1996) and makes people less cautious (Hartley & Shirley, 1977).

During an interrogation, sleep-deprived individuals may use acquiescence as a method of coping with their sleep loss–related cognitive deficits (Blagrove, 1996). Specifically, when people are sleep deprived, they may switch from using an active, cognitive approach to managing their thoughts (Gudjonsson & Clark, 1986) to employing a strategy that seeks to avoid confrontation (Blagrove, 1996).

Notably, although sleep loss does not appear to affect intelligence-related reasoning tasks (Horne, 1988), it does appear to affect logical reasoning tasks (Blagrove, Alexander, & Horne, 1995). The risks associated with these logical reasoning deficits may be further exacerbated by the heightened suggestibility caused by sleep loss (Blagrove, 1996, Blagrove, Cole-Morgan, & Lambe, 1994), particularly the tendency to switch answers in response to negative feedback (Blagrove, Cole-Morgan, & Lambe, 1994). Sleep loss does not reduce people's confidence in the accuracy of their answers, suggesting that sleep-deprived individuals actually internalized the suggested responses, rather than just complying with the requests of authority figures (Blagrove & Akehurst, 2000; Evans & Watson, 1976). High motivation for accuracy

INFO

A prolonged interrogation that results in sleep loss may:

- reduce a suspect's cognitive processing of the *Miranda* warnings;

- interfere with her ability to logically reason about the effects of waiving rights;

- heighten suggestibility to leading questions, particularly after negative feedback;

- and result in the internalization of inaccurate information she provides to police

does not appear to ameliorate the effect of sleep loss on accuracy (Pelham & Neter, 1995).

Police Conduct

PARENTAL PRESENCE

Some states require that a parent be present during interrogation in order to protect the rights of youth and improve the quality of their decision-making around a rights waiver (Cruise, Pitchal, & Weiss, 2008). Additionally, some jurisdictions and even individual police departments choose to have parents present during the questioning of juvenile suspects. Even when no rule exists per se, parental presence may be viewed by judges as an indication that a youth understood and appreciated the rights, that she made an informed decision about waiving rights, and that her waiver was voluntary. However, empirical research on the impact of a parent's presence during interrogation challenges the veracity of these assumptions.

One study, conducted in the 1970s, revealed that most parents who were present during juveniles' interrogations provided little or no advice to their children (see Grisso & Ring, 1979) and may have had no effect on their children's compliance with police requests for information about the alleged offense (Grisso & Pomicter, 1977). Of the 390 interrogations in which parents were present, only about one-third of the parents offered any advice to their children; 60% of these parents encouraged youth to waive their rights to silence and counsel, and about 16% (4% of the total sample) advised against waiving rights (see Grisso & Ring, 1979).

A more recent study suggests that parents continue to fail as protectors of their children's rights during interrogations (Viljoen, Klaver, & Roesch, 2005). Approximately one-quarter of juvenile defendants who were questioned by police reported having had at least one parent present during the interrogation. Forty percent of these youth said that they had not known whether their parents wanted them to make a statement to the police. Of the youth who reported knowing their parents' wishes, 56% said that their parents wanted them to "tell the truth," and 11% indicated that their parents wanted them to deny the offense. No youth reported that their parents advised them to remain silent. Although parents' advice did not significantly predict whether a youth actually remained silent, denied the offense, or confessed (Viljoen, Klaver, & Roesch, 2005), parents' presence during interrogation did not appear to serve the intended protective function.

Grisso and Pomicter (1977) proposed multiple reasons for parents' failure to protect their children's *Miranda* rights: (1) the interrogation setting may be emotionally taxing for both youthful suspects and their parents, and, as a result, parents may be unable to determine what is in their children's best interests; (2) parents might believe that confessions result in outcomes that will be in the best interests of the child; and (3) parents may raise their children to respect and comply with authority figures and to take responsibility for their actions.

STRENGTH OF THE EVIDENCE

During interrogations, police may describe evidence that implicates the suspect in the alleged offense (Inbau, Reid, & Buckley, 2003). Some research suggests that the strength of evidence presented is associated with the likelihood of a rights waiver. For instance, in a vignette-based study (Abramovitch et al. 1995), both school-aged participants and young adults were more likely to say that they would assert the right to silence when the evidence against them was strong than when it was weak. This contrasts, however, with data on the actual behavior of juvenile defendants. Adolescent defendants ages 15 to 17 were more likely to have confessed if they said that the evidence against them had been strong, rather than weak; however, younger defendants' decisions about whether to confess seem to have been unrelated to the strength of the evidence (Viljoen, Klaver, & Roesch, 2005).

In terms of the decision to retain an attorney, school-aged youth were more like to say they would assert the right counsel when the suspect in the vignette was innocent of the alleged offense, but the incriminating evidence against the suspect was strong (Abramovitch et al., 1995).

WORDING OF THE *MIRANDA* WARNING

In the *Miranda* decision, the Court specified the required content of *Miranda* warnings, but did not stipulate the specific wording of the warnings (Oberlander & Goldstein, 2001). As described in the previous chapter, the Court required that the warnings be stated clearly and unequivocally, but each jurisdiction was free to develop its own version. As a result, many versions of the *Miranda* warnings are used, with length, complexity, and reading level varying tremendously across jurisdictions (e.g., Rogers, Harrison, Shuman et al., 2007; Rogers, Hazelwood, Sewell, Shuman et al., 2008).

For instance, one study found that the average warning and waiver was 146 words (ranging from 49 to 547 words) (Rogers, Harrison, Shuman et al., 2007), with an average sentence complexity of 49 (ranging from 12 to 100, on a scale from 0 (not complex) to 100 (very complex)) (Rogers, Hazelwood, Sewell, Harrison, & Shuman, 2008). Reading comprehension level of warnings also varied tremendously across jurisdictions, with Flesch-Kincaid readability levels ranging from grade 3 to 18 Rogers, Harrison, Hazelwood, & Sewell, 2007; Rogers, Hazelwood, Sewell, Shuman et al., 2008). The vocabulary used in *Miranda* warnings varied from requiring a fourth-grade education to a college education (Rogers, Hazelwood, Sewell, Harrison et al., 2008; Rogers, Hazelwood, Sewell, Shuman et al., 2008).

Although these data describe standard, adult versions of *Miranda* warnings, "simplified," juvenile warnings are not necessarily shorter, less complex, or presented at a lower reading level. For instance, one study found that juvenile warnings were an average of 60 words longer than adult warnings and one-half of a grade level more difficult (Rogers, Hazelwood, Sewell, Shuman et al., 2008). The vocabulary content was similar to the adult versions, with many identified words requiring at least a tenth-grade education (Rogers, Hazelwood, Sewell, Shuman et al., 2008). Overall, juvenile *Miranda* warnings seem to be characterized by factors that make them either as difficult (or more difficult) to understand than adult versions.

Despite the recent emphasis on identifying the variability in warnings, little research has evaluated whether complexity affects understanding and appreciation of rights. There is little extant research in this area, and results are inconsistent. One study with mentally disordered defendants from competency to stand trial units at a state hospital found that different versions of the warnings produced different levels of understanding, with mentally disordered defendants demonstrating extensive impairment on all but the simplest *Miranda* warnings (Rogers, Harrison, Hazelwood, & Sewell, 2007). However, other research with juvenile offenders (Messenheimer, Riggs Romaine, Wolbransky, Zelle, Serico, Wrazien, & Goldstein, 2009) and with mentally ill adult inpatients (Cooper & Zapf, 2008) suggested that understanding did not differ between simpler and more complex versions of the warnings. In fact, one study from the 1970s found that juveniles' understanding was actually poorer when simplified warnings were used (Ferguson & Douglas, 1970); this is consistent with Messenheimer and colleagues' (2009) recent findings that juvenile offenders tended to have greater difficulty with some of the simpler warnings than with the more complex versions. Messenheimer and colleagues speculated that shorter, simpler versions may omit some of the critical information from the warnings, thereby depriving the suspect of important details about rights during interrogation.

Thus, although judges may view warning complexity as an important totality of circumstances factor, research has yet to determine whether that assumption is valid. Additionally, from a public policy standpoint, as multiple states and national organizations are working to simplify and standardize *Miranda* warnings (Drogin, 2009), caution should be exercised to establish (1) that "simplified" versions are truly simpler, and (2) that simplification results in improving *Miranda* comprehension, not reducing it.

Research on the Link Between Understanding and Appreciation and Decision to Assert Rights

Research suggests that the decision to assert rights is related to the understanding and appreciation of those rights. In a vignette-based study, youth were more likely to waive rights if they did not adequately understand them (Abramovitch, Higgins-Biss, & Biss,

1993); 90% of school-aged youth who were able to paraphrase a wavier form said that they would not sign it, while 65% of youth who could not explain the form said that they would sign it and waive their rights. In this study, decision-making did not appear to be associated with appreciation of the consequences of waiving rights, probably because so few youth appreciated the rights that there

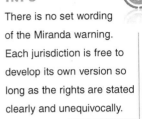

INFO

There is no set wording of the Miranda warning. Each jurisdiction is free to develop its own version so long as the rights are stated clearly and unequivocally.

was not enough variability to detect a relationship. Similarly, in a vignette-based study of male juvenile offenders, the poorer a youths' *Miranda* comprehension, the more likely the youth said he would be to falsely confess to police during interrogation. Notably, however, once age and IQ were taken into account, *Miranda* comprehension was no longer significantly associated with false confessions (Goldstein et al, 2003).

A study of juvenile defendants and the decisions they made during real interrogations supports the findings that rights waivers are associated with *Miranda* comprehension. Among juvenile defendants who were questioned by police, those who waived the right to counsel scored lower on understanding and appreciation of the interrogation warnings than did those youth who asserted this right (Viljoen, Klaver, & Roesch, 2005). There was no relationship between understanding or appreciation and the decision to waive the right to silence. Notably, the requisite legal abilities of *Miranda* understanding and appreciation were a much better predictor of waiver decisions than were measures of more general cognitive abilities.

Research on Assessment Methods

Instruments for Assessing Understanding and Appreciation of *Miranda* Rights

In the 1970s, Grisso created the "Instruments for Assessing Understanding and Appreciation of *Miranda* Rights" as a standardized research tool to examine youths' capacities to understand rights and appreciate the consequences of waiving rights, and to compare these capacities with those of adults. Over the following decades, these instruments were adopted as a specialized forensic assessment tool and, in 1998, they were published (Grisso, 1998). Apparently these instruments were often used in forensic evaluations before 1998, but publication and commercial availability increased their credibility and accessibility as an assessment tool for forensic mental health evaluators examining juvenile and adult defendants' capacities' to have waived *Miranda* rights.

The "Instruments for Assessing Understanding and Appreciation of *Miranda* Rights" consists of four distinct instruments, each of which is designed to assess a different aspect of *Miranda* understanding or appreciation. The content of the instruments and the standardized scoring criteria were created by a panel of lawyers and psychologists.

The four instruments are as follows:

1. Comprehension of *Miranda* Rights (CMR) assesses understanding of the basic meaning of rights by asking examinees to paraphrase the meaning of each right in their own words. Responses are rated as adequate (2 points), questionable (1 point), or inadequate (0 points). Total scores can range from 0 to 8 (up to 2 points for each of the 4 *Miranda* warnings).

2. Comprehension of *Miranda* Rights - Recognition (CMR-R) assesses understanding of the basic meaning of rights, without reliance on verbal expressive abilities, by asking examinees to identify whether preconstructed sentences are the same in meaning to each of the *Miranda* warning statements. Responses are scored as correct (1 point) or incorrect (0 points). Total scores can range from 0 to 12, up to three points for each of the 4 *Miranda* warnings.

3. Function of Rights in Interrogation (FRI) assesses appreciation of the significance of the *Miranda* rights and the consequences of waiving those rights. The examinee is presented with four pictures and

INFO

Grisso's Miranda
Instruments:

- CMR—Comprehension of Miranda Rights

- CMR-R—Comprehension of Miranda Rights - Recognition

- FRI—Function of Rights in Interrogation

- CMV—Comprehension of Miranda Vocabulary

accompanying vignettes about police, legal, and court proceedings. Three subscale scores are calculated to reflect appreciation of the Nature of Interrogation (NI subscale), Right to Silence (RS subscale), and Right to Counsel (RC subscale). Scoring parallels that of the CMR, and total scores can range from 0 to 30 (up to 2 points for each of the 5 items on each of the 3 subscales).

3
chapter

4. Comprehension of *Miranda* Vocabulary (CMV) assesses understanding of six key vocabulary words that were used in the instruments' *Miranda* warnings by asking examinees to define each word. Scoring parallels that of the CMR and FRI, and total scores can range from 0 to 12 (up to 2 points for each of the 6 words).

Research Foundations of the Instruments: Psychometric Data

Research Foundation: Psychometric Properties

The psychometric properties of the instruments that were published in the manual were based on data collected in an extensive study that culminated in 1980, involving offending and nonoffending youth and adults, ages 10 to 50 (Grisso, 1981). Examining the reliability, Grisso (1998) found high internal consistency, inter-rater reliability between trained raters, inter-rater reliability between trained and untrained raters, and high test-retest reliability. Examining validity, Grisso found strong relationships among the instruments and concurrent validity with IQ and age (variables that should be related to understanding and appreciation of rights); content validity was established by having an expert panel create instruments that paralleled the knowing and intelligent criteria of a valid rights waiver. No comparisons were made between instrument scores and external criteria of capacity to waive rights, as judicial decisions about the validity of *Miranda* waivers depend on a totality of circumstances approach, not on performance on just one set of instruments (Grisso, 2004) (see Grisso, 1998, or Goldstein, Condie, and Kalbeitzer, 2005, for detailed data on the psychometric properties of these instruments). An independent investigation (Colwell et al., 2005) further supported the psychometric properties of Grisso's (1998) instruments. This study produced somewhat lower reliability estimates than the original normative data, although reliability remained adequate. Findings on the construct and concurrent validity were strong and consistent with the results of Grisso's (1998) normative study.

Despite the scientific basis and widespread acceptability of the instruments, they have not been without criticism. Rogers and colleagues (2004) reviewed the instruments and criticized them in a published commentary. Some of their criticisms were questionable, reflecting a misinterpretation of the intended use of the instruments, and Grisso (2004) addressed these points directly in his response to Rogers and colleagues' critique. Despite these questionable criticisms, however, Rogers and colleagues (2004) highlighted some specific points that would be valuable for improving the quality of the instruments. Although the instruments were developed under controlled methodology with the common statistical analyses of the time (Frumkin & Garcia, 2003), Rogers and colleagues (2004) suggested that the statistical analyses of the instruments, contemporary norms, and statistical support indicators (e.g., standard errors) needed to be updated and modernized. In addition, they proposed that the assumed, two hypothetical domains of *Miranda* abilities, understanding and appreciation, should be statistically supported through confirmatory factor analysis. These criticisms are being addressed in the revised version of the instruments.

Miranda Rights Comprehension Instruments – II (MRCI-II)

Goldstein, Zelle, and Grisso (in preparation) are revising and updating Grisso's (1998) Instruments. The original instruments were updated for the following reasons: (1) to simplify the language of the wordings to make the instruments more applicable to jurisdictions across the country; (2) to include a fifth warning in the instruments, indicating that suspects can continue to assert their rights at any time, a statement frequently included in *Miranda* warnings; (3) to update the instruments' norms; (4) to update the psychometric properties of the instruments' and conduct additional, more sophisticated analyses that are typical of current times; and (5) to add an additional instrument that begins to assess the voluntariness requirement of a valid *Miranda* wavier (Goldstein, Kalbeitzer, & Condie, 2005). The instruments will be published and available for use in 2010. (For a more detailed summary of the instruments and their development, see Goldstein et al., 2003; Goldstein, Condie, & Kalbeitzer, 2005).

3
chapter

Rogers' Measures

Rogers is in the process of developing a number of scales to assess *Miranda* comprehension and reasoning about waiver decisions. His scales, which were derived from a national sample of *Miranda* warnings, assess comprehension of *Miranda* vocabulary, understanding of the warnings, and reasoning about waiver decisions. The scales are not yet published. (For more detailed summaries of the instruments and their development, see Rogers, Hazelwood, Sewell, Blackwood, Rogstad, & Harrison, 2009; Rogers, Harrison, Hazelwood, & Sewell, 2007).

Research on Assessment Practices - Frequency of Use and Acceptability by Experts

To guide forensic evaluators' selection of assessment tools and courts' reviews of those evaluations, American Board of Professional

Psychology (ABPP) board-certified forensic psychologists were surveyed about the frequency with which they used different tools for forensic evaluations and their opinions about those tools (Lally, 2003). For capacity to waive *Miranda* rights, Grisso's instruments and the Wechsler Adult Intelligence Scale-III (WAIS-III) (Wechsler, 1997) were the only tools recommended by the majority of diplomates. Similarly, a more recent survey revealed that about one-fourth of APA members who listed forensic psychology as an area of interest or practice conduct *Miranda* evaluations; of these practitioners, about 44% reported that they use Grisso's instruments in their evaluations (Ryba, Brodsky, & Shlosberg, 2007). Archer and colleagues (2006), in a survey of AP-LS and AAFP members, found that Grisso's instruments ranked fourth in popularity among tests used in forensic evaluations of adult competency or sanity, more popular than the only criminal responsibility measure and many well-respected measures of competence to stand trial capacities.

Conclusions

To qualify as an expert, forensic mental health practitioners must be knowledgeable about the relevant research in the specialty area. For a case involving a *Miranda* waiver challenge, the expert must be familiar with the empirical data on the totality of circumstances factors relevant to the case, including characteristics of both the defendant and the interrogation. The expert should know and be able to testify about the ways in which the relevant totality of circumstances factors tend to be associated with *Miranda* comprehension deficits and susceptibility to coercive police behaviors. In addition, the expert should be familiar with the available tools for assessing *Miranda* capacities, including the tools' psychometric data and acceptability and use in the field.

APPLICATION

Preparation for the Evaluation | 4

Prior to accepting *any* referral for a forensic mental health assessment, experts must consider a number of issues that could arise. Because no forensic practitioner is an expert in *all* area of forensic assessment, this chapter will help forensic mental heath practitioners decide whether a case involving the assessment of a defendant's capacity to waive *Miranda* rights is a referral that they should accept. In addition, careful consideration of these issues will help experts understand the nature and limits of the specific referral question, clarify their roles in the cases, and help them work with attorneys when conducting these evaluations.

The Referral

Usually, it is the defense attorney who requests an evaluation of defendant's capacity to have waived *Miranda* rights. Typically, the attorney questions whether the client could have knowingly, intelligently, and voluntarily waived the rights required under *Miranda v. Arizona* (1966). At the time of the referral, the expert should discuss with the attorney the precise reasons for the referral.

Nature of the Referral Question

Based upon something the lawyer learned about the defendant's *background and history*, observed about the client's *presentation* (e.g., mentally slow, naive, mentally ill), and/or noted about the *content* of what the client had to say (e.g., about his mental state when the rights were administered, his lack of understanding of the meaning of the rights), the attorney has doubts about the defendant's capacities to have waived *Miranda* rights. Frequently, when the expert asks the attorney for specific reasons why he is questioning his client's capacities to have executed a legally valid waiver, the expert may learn that:

- the client is a juvenile and does not appear to grasp much about the case, including the nature of *Miranda* warnings;

- the client, a juvenile, was questioned without a parent, guardian, or other interested adult present;

- the client, a juvenile, initially refused to speak to the police, but was allowed to speak with his older brother at the police station. After the meeting, the child agreed to talk to interrogators. The older brother may, in the opinion of the lawyer, have pressured the defendant into waiving his rights rather than decided to waive rights on his own;

- the client has a history of mental retardation, psychiatric hospitalization, a learning disability requiring special educational services, or neurological impairment;

- the client denies having received the *Miranda* warnings, and when questioned by the attorney, does not appear to comprehend them;

- the client was born in another country, English is a second language, and the client cannot adequately express himself in English. An interpreter was not provided at the police station and the *Miranda* form was written in English;

- the client claims to have been intoxicated, on drugs, or physically ill (e.g., a diabetic who waived rights 24 hours after the last dose of insulin). The attorney questions whether the defendant "really knew what was going on" at the time of the *Miranda* waiver;

- the client, an adult, tells the attorney that the police said something about "You have the right to be silent," but did not understand the relevance of this or of the other *Miranda* warnings;

- the client claims that the police shouted, threatened, or intimidated him, and he signed the waiver and spoke to interrogators to bring this unpleasant situation to an end; or

- the client claims that promises were made by the police to the effect that if he cooperated and spoke to them about the crime, he could go home that night instead of being held in lock-up. He claims that he was told that cooperation is a positive sign and, as such, there would be little or no punishment. The defendant accepted these promises as realistic and signed the waiver.

Although the referring attorney called to ask the expert, simply, to assess the client's "ability to understand his *Miranda* rights," the specific reasons for the referral question can help structure the evaluation. Reasons for the referral, such as those just described, can alert the expert to issues that might emerge during the assessment, such as young age and cognitive-developmental immaturity, reading problems, attention deficits, low intelligence, active psychosis, problems with judgment and reasoning, altered states of awareness (due to a medical condition or substance abuse), predispositions to feeling overwhelmed or easily threatened by real or imagined threats, or susceptibility to unrealistic promises made by interrogators.

Some lawyers have unrealistic expectations about the opinions experts can ethically offer. For example, an attorney may view his client as highly susceptible to suggestions, believing that the client was coerced into waiving his *Miranda* rights. Although the attorney might want the

BEST PRACTICE

After identifying the nature of the referral question and the attorney's specific concerns about the defendant, you should consider whether:

- the question can be legitimately addressed by a forensic mental health practitioner

- whether you have sufficient expertise in this specific area of forensic practice to conduct the evaluation

BEWARE
Avoid giving
your opinion on whether or
not the defendant was
coerced into waiving
Miranda rights. Your role is
to provide relevant
information to help the judge
make that decision.

expert to provide an opinion about whether the defendant was, in fact, coerced or threatened by interrogators, the expert cannot offer such an opinion; the decision about whether the waiver was coerced is a legal conclusion to be decided by the judge following the suppression hearing in which the expert testifies. Instead, an expert provides relevant information to help the judge make the ultimate decision; in this example, the expert can provide information about whether the defendant possesses characteristics that would increase the likelihood that he would respond to suggestions in a compliant manner, increase his sensitivity to feeling coerced and threatened, and/or increase the probability that he would respond by complying with authority figures' requests to waive *Miranda* rights. Similarly, should an expert testify that a defendant was incapable of providing an intelligent waiver of his *Miranda* rights? We believe that the expert should avoid offering an ultimate opinion if asked this question and instead explain that, based upon the data, the defendant's ability to have provided an intelligent waiver was impaired, citing the nature and level of the impairment.

In sum, the expert should not offer ultimate issue testimony about whether a waiver was provided knowingly, intelligently, and voluntarily. Explaining the limits of potential opinions at the time of the referral can help the attorney develop realistic expectations about the scope of an opinion.

The Decision to Accept the Referral

Although a judge, ultimately, will rule on whether a witness qualifies as an expert, the practitioner should consider whether he has the background, experience, skills, training, or knowledge (*Jenkins v. United States*, 1962; Federal Rules of Evidence, 2001) to accept the case. This is not only a legal question; it is an ethical one, as well, and will be discussed later in this chapter. Some questions the practitioner should ask about himself before accepting the case are:

- Am I familiar with the relevant statutes and case law on the issue of *Miranda* rights waivers?

- Is my knowledge about the specific methodology needed to evaluate this case sufficient?

- Am I familiar with the empirical literature on *Miranda* rights comprehension?

- Do I have the knowledge required to evaluate the defendant, given his background? This question becomes particularly important when the client is from a significantly different background than the evaluator. It is also relevant when instruments commonly used in this area of practice were neither designed for nor normed on this group (this issue will be addressed elsewhere in this chapter).

Attorney's Involvement during the Course of the Evaluation

Evaluations of defendants' capacities to waive *Miranda* rights are retrospective; they focus on a specific time in the past—when the rights were waived or should have been provided to the suspect. By the time the expert conducts the evaluation, a period of time has lapsed since the interrogation—weeks, months, or even years. During this interval, did the defendant acquire additional knowledge about the nature of *Miranda* rights?

Did the Attorney Educate the Client about *Miranda* Rights?

Defendants awaiting trial have considerable time to discuss their cases with fellow inmates. As a result, at the end of each visit with the defendant, the attorney may remind his client, "Don't talk about your case with anyone. Anything you tell someone about your case can be used in court to convict you." Although these instructions are critical to protect the client, the attorney is repeatedly educating the defendant about the fact that anything he says can be used against him in court. Similarly, in discussing the case, the attorney may have educated the client about his rights—the attorney may have told the defendant what the police *should* have told him before questioning and what he *should* have done at the time of interrogation. Furthermore, when informing a client about the purpose of the upcoming evaluation, the attorney may explain why he has concerns about the defendant's understanding of rights, and, in the process, may educate the defendant about those rights. Although such contamination may not be preventable, particularly if the expert has come in long after the interrogation and arrest, it is essential that the expert investigate the nature and extent of the contamination—specifically, the expert should find out what the lawyer has told the defendant about his rights, the risks of self-incrimination, and the nature and purpose of the upcoming evaluation.

Can the Attorney Observe the Evaluation?

At times, defense attorneys ask to observe the assessment. If the prosecutor referred the case, the defense attorney will often ask to be present (because defense attorneys' referrals on this issue are privileged, until a decision is made by the defense to raise the issue formally, prosecutors usually cannot observe the assessment even if they know it is taking place). There is no consensus among experts about whether such a request should be granted.

First, the content of psychological tests is protected by copyright, and there may be legitimate concerns about test security when attorneys observe administration of the instruments. In addition, questions arise about whether the presence of the lawyer may, in some way, affect the outcome of the assessment by altering the defendant's behavior during the evaluation session. In a survey of 160 forensic practitioners, most respondents believed that the presence of a third party during an assessment would negatively affect the evaluation (Shealy, Cramer, & Pirielli, 2008). The researchers emphasized that the issue of whether a defendant is entitled to have an attorney present during the assessment "has not been addressed directly by the U.S. Supreme Court . . . [although] a number of state and federal courts have expressed differing opinions on the issue of attorney presence during forensic evaluations" (pp. 561–562). They noted that in the landmark case *Estelle v. Smith* (1981), the Court indicated that little benefit would be gained by having the lawyer observe the assessment and that the presence of the attorney could possibly harm the assessment process. Hays (2008) emphasized the lack of empirical data on the effects of third-party observations of forensic assessments and noted the need for research on this topic.

Given the inconsistency of case law and the paucity of research, the decision about whether to allow the attorney to be present is, typically, at the expert's discretion. Regardless of whether it is the expert's decision or a court order permitting the lawyer to observe the assessment, the expert should establish ground rules for the evaluation. Limits on the attorney's involvement in the evaluation must be stated, discussed, and clarified in advance of the evaluation.

There is an argument for having the attorney present, at least for the start of the evaluation. Case law (*Estelle v. Smith*, 1981), ethics codes (American Psychiatric Association, 2001; American Psychological Association, 2002), and guidelines on forensic mental health assessments (American Academy of Psychiatry and the Law, 2005; Committee on Ethical Guidelines for Forensic Psychologists, 1991) directly and indirectly address the need to obtain informed consent from clients who are to be forensically evaluated as a result of non–court ordered referrals. For a thorough discussion on the role of the law and ethics in conducting forensic mental health assessments, see the first volume in this series, Heilbrun, Grisso, & Goldstein, 2009; see also Heilbrun, DeMatteo, Marczyk, & Goldstein, 2008.

From a practice perspective, informed consent involves explaining to a client the nature and purpose of the assessment, the expert's unbiased role, that nothing will be considered confidential if a report is written or testimony offered, and that any information relevant to the legal issue in question will be included, even if it may be "harmful" to

BEST PRACTICE

If the defendant's attorney is to be present during the evaluation, be sure to set ground rules. Some suggested ground rules are:

1. the attorney must be an observer, not a participant, in the evaluation

2. the attorney must not advise, interrupt, or speak once the evaluation is underway

3. the lawyer must sit behind the defendant so as not to distract or provide non-verbal (perhaps, unintentional) cues to the client.

the defendant. The defendant must demonstrate his understanding of this information, typically by paraphrasing it. Informed consent requires the client's voluntary consent, not coerced compliance.

Given that the defendant was referred for this forensic evaluation because of potential impairments comprehending a warning about rights, the expert should anticipate problems obtaining informed consent. Most likely, the expert will need to explain, re-explain, and clarify, in simple language, the information needed for informed consent. Notably, if a defendant demonstrates no difficulty providing informed consent, but the expert believes that the defendant's capacities were impaired when he waived his rights during interrogation, the expert needs to offer a reasonable explanation for the discrepancy. Much of the time, however, a defendant will demonstrate difficulty providing informed consent. In such a situation, if the attorney is present at the start of the evaluation, the attorney can authorize that the evaluation continue without the client's informed consent. Consequently, experts should strongly consider making arrangements to have the lawyer present at the beginning of the evaluation, for the informed consent process.

If a referral is court ordered, the judge should clear any communication with the defense attorney or the prosecutor. The judge should indicate in the written and signed order the ground rules of the assessment, such as whether one or both attorneys can be present at the evaluation and whether the evaluation session should be taped. Experts should feel free to make requests and state their preferences and reasons for them, but ultimately, the court makes these decisions.

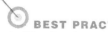

BEST PRACTICE

In *Miranda* waiver cases the defendant may have a hard time understanding the concept of informed consent. It can be helpful to have the defendant's attorney present at the start of the evaluation to aid in the informed consent process.

Autonomy of the Expert vs. Demands of the Attorney

The role of the defense attorney is clear—to defend the client and obtain as short a sentence as possible, using any and all legal and ethical means. As part of this role, the attorney must also protect the client's rights, including the right to remain silent. The forensic mental health expert's role differs dramatically. His main function is to educate the trier of fact, the judge or jury, by providing a thorough, balanced, data-supported opinion, if such an opinion can be reached. This fundamental role difference can create problems when evaluating a defendant's capacities to have waived *Miranda* rights (for a more detailed discussion between these role differences, see Goldstein, 2003).

The defense attorney may ask the expert to limit the scope of questions or refrain from asking his client specific questions. Similarly, the attorney may be willing to provide the expert with some, but not all, records to review. In some cases, these requests may have no impact on the expert's ability to form an informed, unbiased opinion, in which case, it may be acceptable to grant the attorney's requests. However, if specific information (e.g., previous experience with police interrogators) or records (e.g., school records from a juvenile detention center) are required as an integral part of the evaluation, the expert should clearly and assertively inform the attorney about reasons for needing that information. If the attorney insists that these specific areas of inquiry or sources of data are "off limits," the expert is faced with a choice—should he accept the referral? Are there other sources of information available that would provide sufficient information to form an opinion? Alternatively, are the "privileged" sources of data, withheld from the expert, of such a critical nature that the evaluator will not be able to offer an informed opinion following the evaluation? If deprivation of a potentially essential source of information would result in an incomplete or biased data set, the expert should decline the referral. On the other hand, if the information withheld does not seem "essential," the expert can accept the referral and conduct the evaluation; however, in the report and during testimony, the expert should include references to the questions that were not permitted and to the records that were not provided.

Additionally, the expert should briefly note how, if at all, the lack of this information may have limited or affected his opinions.

BEWARE
If the defense attorney does not respond to your requests for certain essential information, you should not accept the referral.

4
chapter

Scheduling the Evaluation

Attorneys who have previously worked with forensic mental health examiners recognize that a credible forensic evaluation requires time and access to multiple sources of information. Experienced lawyers rarely wait until the last minute to contact a forensic mental health expert about a case. Typically, they leave sufficient time to identify an appropriate expert, make fee arrangements, obtain relevant records, and schedule evaluation sessions. They also leave sufficient time to ensure that the expert can interview third parties and, if needed, prepare and submit a written report.

Before accepting a forensic referral, the expert must ask for the date of the hearing. Is there sufficient time to do a thorough, comprehensive job of collecting data, interpreting data, reviewing the relevant literature, writing the report, and preparing for testimony? If not, and if the date of the hearing or trial cannot be changed, then declining the referral is a wise decision.

As will be discussed in chapter 5, more than one interview is typically required. Specialized tests, designed to provide objective information on capacities to waive *Miranda* rights, generally are administered. Objective tests evaluating the defendant's limitations (e.g., low IQ) should be administered, and the expert should explain how these limitations could have impaired the defendant's abilities to knowingly, intelligently, or voluntarily waive his *Miranda* rights. Additional consideration regarding whether malingering or exaggeration may have played a role in the defendant's presentation or performance on other assessment measures may be needed; this may call for specialized measures of response style. Relevant records must be reviewed, and the expert must interview people familiar with the defendant's abilities and limitations that are relevant to comprehending and waiving rights. It is unrealistic to believe that all this can

BEST PRACTICE
Before accepting a referral, make sure there is enough time before the hearing to thoroughly prepare. It is important to provide the attorney with a realistic estimate of the time it will take to conduct interviews and obtain records. If time is an issue, it is best to decline the referral.

be accomplished within a one- or two-week period unless a great deal of information is already available. In some cases, it can take months to obtain the relevant records. It is critical for the expert to present the attorney with a realistic time estimate at the point in the process.

As soon the expert decides to accept the case, an initial appointment should be scheduled. The lawyer should be an active participant in this scheduling, confirming arrangements with both the client and the expert. If the defendant is in custody, the attorney, typically, informs the facility about the meeting, usually in writing, and provides the expert with a copy of the letter. If the expert is not familiar with this particular facility, then the attorney may provide some useful information about official visits (e.g., the physical conditions of the evaluation space, whether there are limitations on time, whether the evaluator can work through scheduled meals, whether there is a"count" involving locking down the facility at certain times).

Location of the Evaluation

The location of the assessment is usually determined by the legal status of the defendant. If the client is detained or incarcerated, scheduling can be straightforward. The facility should be informed, in advance, that the expert will bring tests to the evaluation; otherwise, the introduction of test kits to the facility may not be permitted. The institution should be notified, also in advance, that the expert needs to meet with the defendant in a private, quiet area. Notably, jails and detention centers are neither designed nor run for the comfort and convenience of forensic experts. These institutions are often noisy, lacking in truly private locations, and filled with distractions. Experts should recognize that they are "guests" at the facility, and it is unrealistic to expect a private office. Instead, experts should hope that they are given cubicles with doors that close. Often, these rooms surround general visiting areas. Defendants may be distracted, find it difficult to sustain attention over long time periods of time, and have trouble concentrating. Of course, these difficulties will probably be exacerbated if a defendant has attention problems as

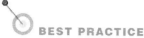

part of his overall diagnostic picture. Although there is little an expert can do to improve the quality of the physical setting for the evaluation, the expert must consider the effects of the conditions when interpreting the data, especially on measures that tap skills like concentration and attention.

If the defendant is not in custody, the forensic mental health expert, in consultation with the attorney, should decide on a location for the evaluation. Options may include the attorney's office, the expert's office, a mental health or court clinic, or the defendant's home. Each has its advantages and disadvantages, such as availability of the defendant and safety.

Particularly when conducting an assessment of a juvenile's *Miranda* waiver capacities or those of an adult who is mentally retarded, there may be distinct advantages to conducting the assessment in the defendant's home. The home-based evaluation will give the expert a flavor of how the defendant lives, and the juvenile or intellectually challenged adult will probably be more comfortable at home than in any other setting. Often, parents or guardians are available, and can be asked to remain at home, so that they also can be interviewed. It is essential to confirm, in advance, whether there is a private, quiet area in the home to conduct the assessment. For safety reasons, conducting assessments of any adult defendants in their homes should be given careful consideration.

Obtaining Collateral Material

An important aspect of best practice in forensic mental health assessment is identifying, obtaining, and relying on third-party information. The process of obtaining relevant records should begin as soon as the referral is accepted. Information acquired directly from the defendant through interviews and testing must be corroborated by others or through record review (Goldstein, 2003;

Grisso, 2003; Heilbrun, Grisso, & Goldstein, 2009; Heilbrun, Warren, & Picarello, 2003; Melton, Petrila, Poythress, & Slobogin, 2007; Otto, Slobogin, & Greenberg, 2007; Simon & Gold, 2004). The *Specialty Guidelines for Forensic Psychologists* (SGFP) (Committee on Ethical Guidelines for Forensic Psychologists, 1991) stress the importance of reviewing such information: "Where circumstances reasonably permit, forensic psychologists seek to obtain independent and personal verification of data relied upon as part of their professional services to the court or a party to a legal proceeding" (p. 662).

Third-party information is a cornerstone of any forensic mental health examination. As defined by Otto, Slobogin, and Greenberg (2007), such data, sometimes referred to as collateral information, "is best described as any information sought or obtained during the course of a forensic examination that does not come directly from the subject of the evaluation" (p. 109). Weissman and DeBow (2003) described the importance of relying on third-party data "for corroborating findings, for ascertaining genuineness, and substantiating allegations, and for testing alternative hypotheses" (p. 42). They also emphasized that following this standard of practice also enhances the overall competence of the assessment (see Otto, Slobogin, & Greenberg, 2007 for a discussion of the laws that govern the use of such information, those factors that affect access to third party information, and practical issues related to obtaining and using such data in an assessment).

Within the context of a psycholegal assessment, where the stakes are high, the defendant's conscious motivation to distort and conceal negative information and to exaggerate and manufacture positive information is obvious. As Rogers (2008a) pointed out, even therapy patients may find it difficult to disclose accurate and complete information within the supportive "context of a psychotherapeutic relationship. The most involved clients may intentionally conceal and distort important data about themselves" (p. 3). In a *Miranda* waiver case, the defendant may realize that if the judge determines that the rights were not validly waived, the confession will be excluded from trial. It is understandable that a defendant

BEWARE
It is critical
to obtain and review
relevant records prior to the
first interview. This will help
you to recognize any
attempts by the defendant to
distort the truth during the
assessment.

might attempt to persuade the expert that *Miranda* comprehension was impaired or that the interrogation was coercive by exaggerating or distorting symptoms. Such misrepresentations are readily seen by mental health professionals as attempts to improve a bad situation (Rogers, Salekin, Sewell, Goldstein, & Leonard, 1998; Rogers, Sewell, & Goldstein, 1994). To address this issue, it is critical that the expert obtain and review relevant records prior to the first appointment. This will allow the expert to recognize and, perhaps, question inconsistencies during the initial evaluation.

Obtaining Signed Releases for Documents

Typically, the attorney is responsible for obtaining copies of a defendant's records. An experienced lawyer usually requests documents before retaining an expert in order to familiarize himself with his client's background, and, potentially, to discover information that will assist in the client's defense. Often, by the time the expert meets with the client, the lawyer will already have had the client sign a number of releases, anticipating that the expert will request additional records. Generally, an agency such as a school or hospital sends the requested records to the attorney; the attorney then copies and sends them to the expert for review.

Categories of Records to Request

Every case is different. Therefore, the list of records to review varies across cases, even if all of the cases involve an evaluation of capacities to waive *Miranda* rights. Nonetheless, there are some general guidelines forensic mental health experts should follow

BEST PRACTICE
When conducting an evaluation of capacity to waive Miranda rights, be sure to request the following:

- Miranda waiver form
- School records
- Mental health records
- Employment records
- Medical records
- Military records

when asking attorneys for specific records in cases involving
Miranda waiver challenges.

ACTUAL *MIRANDA* WAIVER FORM

First and foremost, the expert should request a copy of the
Miranda waiver form that the defendant signed or should have
signed. Although *Miranda v. Arizona* identified the requisite content of the warnings, the specific wording can vary across jurisdictions (*California v. Prysock*, 1981). *Miranda* warnings vary widely
in terms of the number of warnings provided, sentence length,
vocabulary, sentence structure, and reading level (see chapter 3 for
a review of the variations in *Miranda* warning content, language,
and reading level). If the forensic mental health expert is to gauge
the capacity of a defendant to make a knowing and intelligent
waiver of his rights, the expert must question the defendant about
the actual rights administered by police, not about a generic version of those rights.

In some cases, interrogators record the interrogation sessions,
including the administration of the *Miranda* warnings. If such a
recording exists, the expert should obtain and review a copy before
the first meeting with client. In many cases with a recording, the
defendant may have provided a statement to the interrogator
before the recording began and before the reading of the rights
occurred. Although it is important to know whether there was
such a dry run before the "official record" was created, even these
recordings may be highly informative. Review of these recordings
can reveal how quickly the rights were spoken; whether they were
read in a rote, flat manner; whether police provided any explanation of rights; whether the defendant appeared to have paid attention during the administration of the rights, and whether police
gave the defendant an opportunity to indicate whether he understood his rights or had any questions about them.

It is significant that the International Association of Chiefs of
Police (IACP) (April 2004) emphasizes that a suspect's rights prior
to and during interrogation "must be meticulously observed or
any waiver of those rights given by the person being interrogated
is of no effect" (p.1). As such, the IACP Policy Center "calls for

the fullest documentation of the circumstances surrounding interrogations and confessions" (p. 4). The IACP recommends that
each law enforcement agency establish a policy, consistent with the
capabilities of the agency and local case law, to document the location, time, date, and duration of the interrogation; the identity of
those present during the interrogation; the exact wording of the
Miranda warnings given; the suspect's responses to those warnings; and the nature and duration of any breaks in the interrogation for food, drink, rest room visits or other reasons. The IACP
Policy Center recommends that each department select from a
range of methods to document the procedure used, "Handwritten
interrogation logs to computer records to audio or video recording" (IACP, January 2004, p. 2). An expert should request and
review such records after he has accepted the referral.

Defendant's Signed Confession

Unless relevant to the validity or trustworthiness of a confession, it
may not be relevant to review the defendant's signed confession.
Evaluation of a defendant's capacities to have waived his *Miranda*
rights is unrelated to whether or not the defendant committed the
crime. These are two separate issues, as described in chapter 1.
Similarly, it is inappropriate, in terms of the nature and purpose of
the referral, for the expert to ask the defendant for details about
the crime. In fact, it can be extremely irresponsible for an evaluator
to ask the defendant for such information. In some jurisdictions,
evidentiary law may not prohibit the introduction of the defendant's statement about the crime; such information could be used
against the defendant as evidence of guilt. In such circumstances,
if the defendant provides details about the crime, he may provide
a second, independent confession that could
replace the one, at issue, that the judge may
suppress. This caution represents a substantial distinction in practice from evaluations
of a defendant's mental state at the time of
the crime, evaluations that depend heavily
on the defendant's report of details about
the crime.

BEWARE
You should
never ask the defendant
for details of the crime.
They are not relevant
to the evaluation of the
defendant's capacities
to waive his *Miranda*
rights.

OTHER CATEGORIES OF RECORDS

Many cases in this area of forensic mental health assessment involve claims that the defendants have low IQ scores, mental health problems, reading deficits, ADHD, or other impairments that may have resulted in previous special education services. The records may describe the nature of special education services, list the defendants' specific areas of difficulty, and identify steps needed to remediate the problems. The defendant's grades, academic history, and scores on standardized tests (intelligence tests, measures of reading and writing) may be relevant. Therefore, it is critical that the expert review school records. Records may confirm the existence of claimed or suspected diagnoses prior to the interrogation, which, in part, can address the frequently raised issue of possible malingering or exaggeration.

In addition, many defendants who are evaluated for their capacities to waive *Miranda* rights have emotional problems that may interfere with their attention spans, abilities to make reasoned decisions, and overall judgment. If a defendant has been in psychotherapy, seen as an outpatient at a clinic, or been psychiatrically hospitalized, those records should be requested and reviewed as soon as possible.

Despite significant impairments, the defendant may have a history of employment, and the expert should review employment records and, potentially, speak with current or former supervisors. Like many people, defendants may be embarrassed by their low levels of functioning and may make misleading claims about their work. For example, a defendant may have indicated that he worked, very successfully, delivering lunch orders to customers. However, record review and an interview with the owner might reveal that the defendant consistently got lost when making deliveries, despite specific directions and repeated visits to these same locations, and the defendant was unable to reliably make change for customers.

MEDICAL RECORDS

If the defendant has received treatment for a condition that might serve as a partial or complete explanation for the impairments found in *Miranda* rights comprehension, treatment and hospital records should be requested as soon as possible. Loss of consciousness, history of hyperactivity, or head injury may all be relevant factors to be considered, documented, and corroborated.

MILITARY RECORDS

Although military records will rarely reveal a history of intellectual limitations that would serve to explain deficits in the capacity to waive *Miranda* rights (unless the defendant suffered brain injury while in the service), a history of exposure to traumatic events, not limited to a formal diagnosis of Posttraumatic Stress Disorder, could explain a defendant's reaction when questioned by authority figures. When under stress (i.e., when considered a suspect in a crime and questioned by trained interrogators), a defendant may quickly feel threatened—both physically and emotionally—regardless of how realistic such threats may be. Thus, military records may provide relevant information when a lawyer raises the issue of the voluntariness of a *Miranda* waiver assessment, and these records should be requested and reviewed as part of the evaluation.

Third Party Interviews

As previously discussed, people familiar with the defendant may have information that can corroborate or refute claims the defendant made about his history, limitations, or conditions that might have affected his capacity to have waived *Miranda* rights. In preparation for the assessment, the expert should ask the referring attorney to identify third parties who may later be interviewed to corroborate information provided by the defendant. These people may be able to provide additional insight, not only about the defendant's cognitive or emotional impairments, but also about the client's mental state close to the time of the waiver.

Special Ethical Concerns

As discussed in detail in the first volume of this series, *Foundations of Forensic Mental Health Assessment* (Heilbrun, Grisso, & Goldstein, 2009), professional ethics sources contribute substantially to the best-practice standards in forensic mental health assessment.

"The Ethical Principles of Psychologists and Code of Conduct" (Ethics Code), authored by the American Psychological Association (2002), applies to *all* psychologists, regardless of specialization. Similarly, the *Principles of Medical Ethics with Annotation Especially Applicable to Psychiatry* (American Psychiatric Association, 2001), applies to *all* psychiatrists, regardless of practice area. Because such codes are purposefully worded in somewhat general terms to apply to a broad range of situations, other documents—guidelines—were created to address specific areas of practice, including forensic mental health practice by psychologists and psychiatrists.

"The Specialty Guidelines for Forensic Psychologists" (SGFFP) (Committee on Ethical Guidelines for Forensic Psychologists, 1991), authored by a committee of members of the American Board of Forensic Psychology (ABFP) and the American Psychology-Law Society (AP-LS; Division 41 of the APA), is an aspirational model that applies the Ethics Code to forensic situations; currently, the SGFFP is being revised. The "Ethics Guidelines for the Practice of Forensic Psychiatry", developed by the American Academy of Psychiatry and the Law (AAPL) (American Academy of Psychiatry and the Law, 2005), serves a similar purpose—applying the more general ethical principles of psychiatry to forensic settings. The significant differences between the roles of treating professional and forensic mental health evaluator (Appelbaum, 1997, Appelbaum & Gutheil, 2007; Goldstein, 2003; Greenberg & Shuman, 1997; Lipsitt, 2007; Weissman & DeBow, 2003) are so important that the expert must be very familiar with these guidelines; attending to the details of these guidelines can also help the expert reduce or eliminate embarrassing questions that may arise during cross-examination. This section considers significant ethical issues that may arise when evaluating a defendant's capacity to have validly waived *Miranda* rights.

Competence of the Evaluator

Expertise in forensic mental health assessment is not generic. Each type of psycholegal evaluation requires specific knowledge in order to perform the assessment in an ethical, competent fashion. Melton and colleagues (2007) stressed that experts should have "specialized knowledge about relevant legal standards and issues, the technology of various forms of forensic assessment, and the effects of various dispositions (p. 103)." In addition, when conducting any type of forensic assessments, the examiner must be aware of the constitutional rights of the examinee and respect those rights, as required by law.

In his landmark book, *Evaluating Competencies: Forensic Assessments and Instruments*, Grisso (1986) presented common criticisms of forensic mental health evaluations. He wrote that when major difficulties arise, it is often due to:

- *Ignorance* of the evaluator and *irrelevance* of elements of the opinions,

- *Intrusion* of the evaluator into matters that should be left to the trier of fact, and,

- *Insufficiency* of data to support opinion

Competence in conducting *Miranda* rights waiver evaluations must involve a thorough awareness of the goals, scope, limitations, and methodology of these specialized assessments. Such familiarity should reduce the likelihood of the common pitfalls Grisso identified.

Competence requires practicing within the boundaries of one's expertise. The Ethics Code (American Psychological Association, 2002, Section 2.01) specifies that these boundaries are based on the "education, training, supervised experience, consultation, study, or professional experience" of the psychologist. Psychologists who assume forensic roles must "become reasonably familiar with the judicial or administrative rules governing their roles" (Section 2.01(f)), another facet of competence, according to the Ethics Code. In addition, psychologists must possess "an understanding of factors associated with age, gender, gender identity, race, ethnicity, culture, national origin, religion, sexual orientation, disability, language or socioeconomic status . . . to ensure competence of services. . . ." (Section 2.01(b)). For instance, if the defendant is a juvenile, the evaluator should have expertise "in the patterns of development, psychopathology, and offending that are typical in juvenile justice settings" (Kruh & Grisso, 2009, p. 89). The American Psychological Association (1993) also authored guidelines for providing services to culturally diverse populations.

According to the SGFFP (Committee on Ethical Guidelines for Forensic Psychologists, 1991), competence involves the recognition that, when testifying in court, experts have factual bases for their competence, the "knowledge, skill, experience, training, and education" that qualify them as experts on the specific area of testimony" (Section III B). Because of their involvement in the legal system, it is expected that "Forensic psychologists are responsible for a fundamental and reasonable level of knowledge and understanding of the legal and professional standards that govern their participation as experts in legal proceedings" (Section III C).

An ethical concern can arise in *Miranda* waiver evaluations if the psychologist's opinions may be affected by his concerns that the judge will suppress a statement based on the expert's testimony—if the judge excludes a confession, the prosecutor may need to drop the case or, if tried without the confession, the defendant may be freed, despite having committed a horrendous crime. The *SGFFP* cautions that "Forensic psychologists recognize that their own personal values, moral beliefs, or personal and professional relationships with parties to a legal proceeding may interfere with their ability to practice competently. Under such circumstances, forensic psychologists are obligated to decline participation or limit their assistance in a matter consistent with professional obligations" (Section III E). If the expert is significantly troubled by the possibility that a potentially violent defendant will be freed on what he considers to be "a legal technicality," the practitioner should decline to conduct this type of forensic mental health assessment. Personal biases may interfere with or color data interpretation and the opinions reached, affecting the objectivity of the assessment.

Human Relationships

Section 3.04 of the Ethics Code (American Psychological Association, 2002) requires psychologists to "take reasonable steps to avoid harming their clients/patients . . . and to minimize harm where it is foreseeable." In addition, Section 3.07 addresses the need, at the outset of a professional relationship, to clarify the nature of the relationship, including roles,

4
chapter

BEWARE
Take heed of any personal bias or preconceived notions that may interfere with your objectivity in a particular case.

the possible "uses of the services provided or the information obtained, and the fact that there may be limits to confidentiality." This is considered to be part of the informed consent process; the Ethics Code (Section 3.10) requires that informed consent be obtained, except in those circumstances that do not require informed consent, such as a court ordered assessment. The code states that language appropriate to the client be used so that it is "understandable to that person" (Section 3.10(a)), and, if the person cannot provide informed consent, the expert can take a number of alternative actions to protect the defendant's rights, such as obtaining permission from someone who is legally authorized to provide it, obtaining informed assent from the examinee (i.e., an agreement to participate that does not meet the legal threshold of informed consent but that is as informed as possible given the examinee's limitations), and actively considering the client's best interests and preferences (Section 3.10(b)). As discussed earlier, this principle is especially relevant when working with defendants suspected of having difficulty understanding their *Miranda* rights.

Similarly, the SGFFP, Section IV. E. (Committee on Ethical Guidelines for Forensic Psychologists, 1991), emphasizes the need to inform clients of their legal rights, the nature and purpose of the assessment and of the methods to be used, and who has retained the expert. In addition, this document states that the client or the attorney should provide informed consent (unless the assessment is court ordered) (Section IV. E. 1.) and the evaluation should not be conducted without legal notice to the lawyer (Section IV. E. 2). Also, only information relevant to the legal matter for which informed consent was obtained should be provided in a report or in testimony unless there is waiver by the client or the attorney to allow for other legal uses of the findings (Section IV. E. 3).

Privacy and Confidentiality

Issues regarding privacy and confidentiality relate directly to informed consent. The Ethics Code (American Psychological Association, 2002) requires that the psychologist explain the foreseeable uses of the product of the assessment (e.g., the report and testimony) to the examinee (Section 4.01 (a)), and "only information germane to the purpose" of the evaluation be communicated in that product. Similarly, the *SGFFP* (Committee on Ethical Guidelines for Forensic Psychologists, 1991) states that even though the client's confidentiality may be limited, "the forensic psychologist makes every effort to maintain confidentiality with regard to any information that does not bear directly upon the legal purpose of the evaluation (Section V. C)." Although defendants who are to be evaluated because of questions related to the validity of their *Miranda* waivers may have difficulty grasping this information, the expert must make a concerted effort to ensure comprehension. Failing adequate comprehension, authorization to continue with the assessment must be provided by the attorney, unless the evaluation was court ordered.

Record Keeping

The Ethics Code (American Psychological Association, 2002) stresses the importance of written records in *all* areas of psychological practice. Section 6.01 of the code discusses the importance of documentation and maintenance of records, citing a number of reasons, including the need to "facilitate provision of services later by them or other professionals . . . [and to] ensure compliance with the law." The SGFFP (Committee on Ethical Guidelines for Forensic Psychologists, 1991) applies this general principle to forensic mental health assessments. Specifically, forensic psychologists are obligated to document and offer "all data that form the basis for their evidence or services. The standard to be applied to such documentation or recording anticipates that the detail and quality of such documentation will be subject to reasonable judicial scrutiny" (Section VI. A.). The *SGFFP* emphasizes that the standard for documentation in this specialized area of practice is *higher* than the standard in the general practice of clinical psychological practice.

When conducting a forensic mental health assessment of a defendant's capacity to have validly waived *Miranda* rights, the expert must keep thorough notes of each interview, including how informed consent was obtained and questions asked of the defendant. Keeping thorough records in the context of forensic evaluations involves documenting, verbatim, the questions put to the defendant and his exact answers, during both interviews and testing. This requires the expert to write quickly, slow the respondent down when necessary, and judiciously keep notes that will serve as the basis of the written report and testimony. In addition, for better or worse, in the interest of fairness, detailed notes will serve to inform the opposing lawyer when preparing to cross-examine the expert.

Verbatim recording is particularly important in *Miranda* waiver evaluations. When a defendant attempts to explain the meaning of a specific *Miranda* right, his choice of one word over another can convey subtle shades of comprehension, information that can prove invaluable to both the expert in writing the report, and to the judge when deciding the legal issue before the court. Paraphrasing a defendant's responses or retroactively creating records based on memory of what was said is a serious violation of both ethical principles and the standard of practice.

The Record Keeping Guidelines (American Psychological Association, 2007) mostly focus on clinical records, but they do emphasize that a number of considerations should enter into the decision about the level of detail that should be included in the records; the purpose of the evaluation is certainly one of those considerations. We recommend that, consistent with the SGFFP (Committee on Ethical Guidelines for Forensic Psychologists, 1991), records of *Miranda* waiver evaluations be verbatim notes of what was said during each assessment session. The Record Keeping Guidelines recommend that psychologists should consider maintaining records "until seven years after the last date of service for adults or until three years after a minor reaches the age of majority, whichever is last" (p. 999). However, because of the unique nature of forensic mental health assessment, Heilbrun, Grisso, and Goldstein (2009) "recommend that in forensic contexts, psychologists should consider retaining full records for a longer period of time" (p.69). This is

BEST PRACTICE

Keeping verbatim records is particularly important in *Miranda* waiver evaluations where the defendant may have problems with comprehension. Be sure to take detailed notes and avoid paraphrasing defendant responses.

especially true with *Miranda* rights waiver assessments, where many defendants are minors at the time of their initial evaluations. Some defendants may reoffend in the future, and interview notes and test data may be of value long after seven years. Similarly, appeals can be filed after many intervening years, even decades.

Assessment

The psychological assessment section of the Ethics Code (American Psychological Association, 2002) is particularly relevant to the practice of forensic psychology. Section 9.01 requires that opinions reached by psychologists, including those offered during testimony, be based "on information and techniques sufficient to substantiate their findings." Assessment instruments should have established reliability and validity "for use with members of the population tested" (Section 9.02 (b)). If adequate psychometric properties have not been established with the relevant population(s) (e.g., female, African American), the expert must describe how this limits the results and conclusions of testing. In interpreting test results, The *Ethics Code* requires psychologists to consider any factors, including "situational, personal, linguistic, and cultural differences that might affect psychologists' judgments or reduce the accuracy of their interpretations" (Section 9.06).

The SGFFP (Committee on Ethical Guidelines for Forensic Psychologists, 1991) indicates that psychologists should select methods and procedures for conducting forensic mental health assessments "consistent with accepted clinical and scientific standards" (Section VI. A.). As discussed earlier in this chapter, because of the unique nature of the field, critical data, including hearsay evidence, should be corroborated if used as a basis for opinions. If hearsay evidence is uncorroborated, it should be presented as such.

Many defendants referred for evaluations of their capacities to have waived *Miranda* rights are from minority populations, and English may be a second language. They often come from diverse cultural backgrounds. As such, performance on tests that were normed on other populations may not be directly interpretable—the expert may need to qualify scores, explain performance patterns, and clearly present limits on the interpretability and applicability of results. Despite the extra caution required of the expert when interpreting data and presenting findings, this does *not* mean that defendants from multicultural groups cannot be administered standardized tests (e.g., intelligence tests). Instead, the expert must describe the potential effects of a defendant's background on test results in the written report and during testimony.

When evaluating a defendant's capacities to have executed a valid *Miranda* rights waiver, the use of culturally valid and reliable assessment tools may not be as significant an issue as it might first appear. The Ethics Code (American Psychological Association, 2002, Section 9.02 (c)) states "Psychologists use assessment methods that are appropriate to an individual's language preference and competence, *unless the use of an alternative language is relevant to the assessment issues*" (emphasis added). In *Miranda* rights waiver cases, the actual waiver may have been presented in English, even if the suspect was not fluent in English. Having an interpreter translate the rights into the defendant's native language would likely distort the assessment of the client's comprehension of the rights as they were originally presented at the time of the waiver. Using an English-based assessment instrument, which puts the defendant at a disadvantage because of language and cultural factors, may actually mirror his experience at the time of interrogation.

Conclusions

A referral to evaluate a defendant's capacity to execute a valid waiver of his *Miranda* rights requires consideration of many factors, such as clarifying the reasons for referral with the attorney, determining the scope of the evaluation, establishing a working relationship with the lawyer, and determining what the defendant may have learned about his rights since the time of the waiver. As soon as he accepts a case, the expert should request relevant records, especially a copy of the waiver form used in the jurisdiction in which the defendant was arrested. The expert should also identify third parties he may want to interview. In addition, he should consider ethical issues relevant to forensic assessment generally and *Miranda* waiver evaluations in particular. These include professional competence, confidentiality, the need to obtain informed consent, assessment methodology, and record keeping.

4
chapter

Data Collection | 5

This chapter describes the sources of data that experts should consider when conducting evaluations of defendants' capacities to have waived *Miranda* rights. Typically, such sources include interviews of the defendant; administration of traditional tests, forensic assessment instruments designed specifically for this purpose, forensically relevant instruments (e.g., tests of malingering of symptoms associated with mental retardation, memory loss, or psychosis); and collateral information (e.g., written documents, third-party interviews). Decisions about which information to rely upon, how much weight to give each source of information, and how to interpret the obtained data must be made on a case-by-case basis.

Interviewing the Defendant

In most cases involving this psycholegal question, more than one interview session is needed. Multiple sessions are usually needed because:

- The quantity of historical information to be obtained from the defendant is extensive;
- The defendant must be questioned in detail about the circumstances of the arrest, how the rights were administered, and her comprehension of those rights;
- Psychological testing is typically required; and
- After scoring the tests, reviewing the results, and examining third-party information, additional

questions may arise. The need for more testing may be indicated, and some previously obtained information may require clarification.

There are many goals of forensic interviews in *Miranda* cases:

- Acquire a detailed background history from the defendant;
- Assess the defendant's mental status (including the ability to provide informed consent);
- Observe the defendant's behavior and approach to tasks;
- Identify additional sources of corroborative information (e.g., records, other people to interview);
- Evaluate the defendant's accuracy, honesty, and openness when reporting historical data by comparing this information to corroborative information; and
- Obtain the defendant's version about how the confession was obtained and her capacities to have comprehended and voluntarily waived the rights.

Obtain Informed Consent

As discussed previously, from both legal and ethical perspectives, the forensic mental health expert must attempt to obtain informed consent from the defendant; if it is a court ordered evaluation, the expert need only provide notification of purpose. It is essential to document carefully how informed consent was obtained. If informed consent could not be obtained because of the defendant's limitations, the process should still be documented, capturing the defendant's difficulties comprehending the information she was told.

Obtain Relevant Background History

Any forensic assessment requires a detailed understanding of the defendant's background.

In *Miranda* waiver cases, the relevant history has a particular focus: the potential relationship between prior historical events and

INFO

Relevant areas to be covered in *Miranda* cases generally include:

- Parental history and methods of discipline
- Background of siblings
- Educational history
- Military service
- Vocational history
- Marital status
- Relevant medical conditions and prior mental health treatment
- Alcohol and drug use
- Prior arrests and convictions
- Other areas of inquiry related to general comprehension, reasoning skills, judgment, and decision-making

the capacity of the defendant to have executed a valid waiver of Constitutional rights. Some examples of how historical factors could affect waiver capacities follow.

PARENTAL HISTORY AND METHODS OF DISCIPLINE

Is there a parental history of mental retardation, Attention Deficit Hyperactivity Disorder (ADHD), learning disability, or psychosis? How was the defendant punished? Is there a history of acquiescence to authority? Data from these and related questions may explain problems with capacity to comprehend the rights or to have voluntarily waived them. For instance, an adolescent raised in a home requiring strict obedience to authority (and harsh punishment if obedience is not provided) may be somewhat predisposed to accepting demands made by interrogators in an unquestioning, uncritical manner, conforming to their requests to waive rights and provide confession.

SIBLINGS' HISTORY

Is there a familial history of mental retardation, learning disability, ADHD, or psychosis? How consistent is the defendant's educational level with that of her siblings? Data from this area of inquiry may suggest a familial basis for a number of disorders.

EDUCATIONAL HISTORY

Was the defendant held back in school? How far did she go in school? Did the defendant need or receive special educational services? Did the defendant have an individualized educational plan (IEP)? This may reveal long-standing problems in such areas as reading, listening comprehension, oral expression, general comprehension, attention, concentration, or impulsivity.

MILITARY SERVICE

Did the defendant serve in the military? How did her career progress while in the service? What problems were encountered and what was the nature of the discharge? Questions about this topic may reveal such information as relationships with authority figures (e.g., acquiescence, deference, conformity), problems grasping the nature of tasks, and performance in high-risk and high-pressured situations.

VOCATIONAL HISTORY

Has the defendant been employed? Who completed the job applications? What positions did she hold and what is her version of the responsibilities involved, her performance, and reasons for leaving jobs? Has she ever applied or qualified for Social Security Disability payments? This employment information may contribute to an expert's opinion that the defendant has been limited in many ways, having difficulty finding a job, performing tasks in an independent, satisfactory manner, and understanding responsibilities. Questions about employment history may also reveal whether others have reported problems in her comprehension, judgment, independent functioning, and employability. As with educational history, historic problems with employment often are documented in records or can be described by neutral, third parties; this, in turn, can provide convincing evidence of long-standing problems that predated the arrest and waiver in question.

MARITAL STATUS AND RELATIONSHIP HISTORY

Does the defendant live with someone or has she in the past? With whom did she live and what was that person like (e.g., level of education; employment)? How long did the relationship(s) last and why did it(they) end? What were the sources of conflict? Such questions may produce relevant information about the defendant's social maturity, interaction patterns when in stressful situations, and ways of handling responsibility. Such information may shed some light on how the defendant might have responded to the stress associated with an interrogation and the defendant's ability to resist acquiescing to the demands of the interrogators.

RELEVANT MEDICAL CONDITIONS AND PRIOR MENTAL HEALTH TREATMENT

Are there any prior medical conditions, including past hospitalization for conditions that might explain intellectual limitations; problems focusing attention; or difficulties with judgment, comprehension, or memory? A history of head trauma, brain dysfunction, or diabetes (not under control at the time of interrogation) may explain impairments at the time the defendant waived her *Miranda* rights. Is there a history of mental health treatment? What were the symptoms? Was the defendant prescribed psychotropic medication for this condition, and was she taking it, as prescribed, around the time of interrogation? This information may be relevant to the defendant's claims of difficulty comprehending the rights when they were administered. Certain medications, particularly if recently prescribed, may interfere with concentration or result in extreme sleepiness, a state that could interfere with active processing of information and heighten suggestibility. Failure to take psychotropic medication may be associated with a return of symptoms that produce difficulty focusing attention, accurately understanding what is being said, and forming reasoned judgments—such as a decision that is in one's best interests.

USE OF ALCOHOL AND DRUGS

What is the defendant's substance-use history? Did the defendant consume alcohol or use drugs before her arrest and interrogation? How long before the rights were administered were substances last used? Intoxication may explain a defendant's confusion, lack of focus, suggestibility, and poor decision-making. If a defendant was inebriated or high to the point that she could not make a knowing, intelligent, and voluntary waiver of her rights, the judge should consider the waiver invalid and suppress the incriminating statement. It is irrelevant in a *Miranda* waiver case whether the defendant voluntarily ingested the alcohol or drugs—the only question at issue in a suppression hearing is whether the defendant had the capacities to meet the legal criteria for a valid waiver. The reason for the failure to provide a valid waiver is not required—it only serves as a basis to help the court understand the reasons behind the failure and to provide credibility for the alleged failure.

PRIOR ARRESTS AND CONVICTIONS

Was the defendant arrested before, either as a juvenile or an adult? What previous experiences did the defendant have with the juvenile and criminal justice systems? Had she been provided her rights before? Had she been interrogated previously? If so, what happened and why? It is essential to obtain a history of the defendant's previous exposure to the *Miranda* warnings and prior contact with interrogators. If a defendant had exercised her *Miranda* rights during a prior interrogation, the evaluator will need to explain why the rights were waived in the present arrest. Yet this should be considered in the broader context of research evidence indicating that experience with the police (e.g., previous arrests) does not seem to be associated with better *Miranda* rights comprehension (see chapter 3 for a thorough discussion of research findings on this relationship).

OTHER AREAS OF INQUIRY

Here, we are referring to case-specific issues that *may* be relevant—such characteristics as a defendant's reasoning, judgment, and decision-making abilities that may contribute to having the capacities needed to provide a meaningful waiver of rights. What television shows does the defendant watch, and can she describe their overall plot? What newspapers and magazines does the defendant read, and can she describe an article that she found interesting? What is the defendant's understanding of major events that are currently in the news? Does she hold a driver's license, and how many times did she take the test until she passed? Could she read the driver's manual? Did she pass a nonverbal test to get a learner's permit? Does the defendant have a bank or checking account, and who balances the checkbook? Although some questions may not produce relevant information, others may yield very revealing information that provides data relevant to the defendant's capacities to have waived her *Miranda* rights.

Defendant's Rendition of Events Surrounding the Rights Waiver

As is the case in most criminal forensic evaluations, especially those that are retrospective in nature, the defendant is usually the primary source of information about her mental state and functioning at the time of the event in question. As such, during the interview, the forensic mental health professional must ask the defendant about her mental state; the expert must also ask for her recollections of her comprehension of the rights when they were presented and her abilities to have executed a rights waiver at that time.

During the interviews, the expert should ask the defendant directly about a number of areas. These include:

- her recollections of her mental state at the time of the waiver;

- her comprehension of the *Miranda* rights at the time of the waiver;

- the conditions under which the rights were administered (e.g., loud location where she had trouble hearing interrogators; busy room where she had trouble focusing on the information police provided);

- descriptions of the behavior of the interrogators (e.g., threats or promises that may have been made, tone of voice; interactions with each other); and

- any other factors that may have affected her comprehension of rights (e.g., physical illness or a drug-withdrawal reaction that interfered with her ability to focus on the rights) or her ability to have made a voluntarily decision to waive her rights

5
chapter

(e.g., common police brutality in culture of origin; physical threats from fellow gang members if she did not confess).

As discussed in detail in chapters 1, 2, and 3, judges use the totality of circumstances approach to determine the validity of a *Miranda* waiver. This approach requires consideration of the characteristics of the suspect, as well as the circumstances under which the suspect waived the rights and the provided inculpatory statement. Thus, the judge may consider a wide range of intellectual and personality characteristics, and a comparably wide range of situational variables, as a basis for the legal opinion.

It is critical that the expert ask the defendant detailed questions about the interrogation and waiver in question. How many times did police interrogate her and did they present the *Miranda* rights each time? Where did each interrogation take place? At what time of day or night did questioning occur? Was the defendant tired or sleep deprived? Did the defendant's comprehension of rights improve over the course of the repeated interrogations? Did family or friends provide advice between interrogations, and, if so, what was the nature of that advice? Did she feel coerced or threatened by family members, and what effect did that have on her decision to waive her rights and speak with the police? Were any or all interrogation sessions recorded?

Defendants may claim to have been questioned, with or without having received their rights, prior to the recorded interrogation. That is, was there a "dry run" of the questioning and confession before the video cameras were turned on? What happened during the unrecorded interrogation session or sessions? Did the police present the defendant with her rights prior to the "dry run?" Did the police suggest or promise more lenient treatment if the defendant waived her *Miranda* rights and confessed to the crime?

Other than the interrogators who may not be willing to be interviewed and who may also distort what occurred behind the doors of the interrogation room, the defendant is the only source of this information. However, the defendant might be inclined to exaggerate or fabricate information to suggest that the waiver was not voluntary and that the confession should be excluded from trial. In addition, the defendant's memory of the events surrounding police questioning may be genuinely distorted due to the passage of time between the interrogation and the expert's assessment.

Although the expert must obtain the defendant's recollection of the events surrounding the *Miranda* waiver, the expert must consider the trustworthiness of these data within the context of their source. Unfortunately, interrogators often avoid providing experts with detailed information about the circumstances surrounding the waiver, especially if the expert was retained by the defense. If the interrogators do speak with the expert and offer testimony in court, they, too, have an identifiable motive to distort what may have occurred.

> **BEWARE**
> It is important to consider that the defendant may exaggerate or lie when describing the circumstances of her interrogation. Also, the defendant's memory of the interrogation may be genuinely distorted due to the amount of time that has passed since she was questioned by police.

Defendant's Comprehension of *Miranda* Rights

As discussed previously, before seeing the defendant, the expert should obtain and review a copy of the actual waiver of rights form the defendant signed. If no signed waiver exists, the expert should bring to the examination session a copy of the rights that police read to the defendant. No general agreement exists about how an expert should proceed when questioning the defendant about her rights. We provide a suggested strategy in the paragraphs that follow, but, because the *totality of circumstances* surrounding each

> **BEST PRACTICE**
> You may wish to use the following suggested strategy for questioning the defendant about his rights:
>
> 1. use open-ended, nonleading questions to ask the defendant about rights
> 2. review the signed *Miranda* waiver form, if one exists
> 3. ask the defendant to read the form aloud
> 4. administer Grisso's *Instruments for Assessing Understanding and Appreciation of Miranda Rights*

5 chapter

case differs, the expert should decide on the specifics of how best to proceed with the evaluation. The expert should be prepared to explain this decision if asked in court.

In most cases, we suggest that the expert begin asking broadly about rights, using open-ended, nonleading questions. For instance, the expert can assess the defendant's ability to spontaneously produce information about rights by asking, "What did the police say to you when you were arrested?" or "What were the police supposed to say to you when you were arrested?" If the defendant seems puzzled, does not understand the question, or provides information not directly related to the rights (e.g., "They told me to get in the cop car"), the expert may offer a nonleading prompt, such as, "I'm guessing you've watched TV and seen movies in which someone was arrested. What do police say to the person they're arresting?" If the defendant continues to provide irrelevant information, the examiner might consider asking the defendant more directly about her rights, saying something like "When the police arrest someone, they're supposed to tell them their rights—what are those rights?" If the defendant offers little to no response, the expert may want to push the defendant somewhat. For example, the expert may say, "Most people can remember some of the rights police are supposed to tell a suspect. I'm sure you can think of some." If the defendant recalls some, but not all of the rights, she should be asked to try to think of additional rights that police are supposed to present. The evaluator should then ask the defendant to explain the meaning of each right that she spontaneously recalls and ask her to clarify any information that is unclear.

Next, the expert should review the actual *Miranda* rights from the jurisdiction in which the waiver took place. Before showing the defendant a copy of the signed *Miranda* waiver form, the expert should ask the defendant whether she had been given a form to sign and, if so, whether she signed it. If the defendant claims that she never saw a *Miranda* waiver form, but the expert has one bearing the defendant's signature (or, in some cases an "X"" because she does not speak English or cannot print or write her name), the expert should ask the defendant about this discrepancy.

After any discrepancies are clarified about what was presented at the time of the interrogation, the expert should ask the defendant to read the waiver form aloud, right by right. If no waiver form exists, the expert should ask the defendant to read a copy of the *Miranda* rights used in the jurisdiction in which the arrest took place. This right-by-right review will provide some information about the defendant's ability to read the form; this information should be compared to test results and records that more objectively measure reading ability. If the defendant is unable to read the form, the expert can read it aloud to her. After each right is read aloud, either by the defendant or expert, the defendant should be asked to paraphrase the right.

Finally, if the forensic mental health evaluator is concerned about whether the defendant was capable of providing a knowing and intelligent waiver of rights, the evaluator should administer Grisso's *Instruments for Assessing Understanding and Appreciation of Miranda Rights* (Grisso, 1998b, and see chapter 3 for a detailed description of these instruments,). As discussed later in this chapter, the instruments offer a structured, objective approach to evaluating a defendant's *Miranda* comprehension. In addition, the instruments were normed and, therefore, also provide information about how the defendant's comprehension compares to that of other individuals of similar ages and with similar IQ scores.

At times, defendants will explain that while they *now* understand the meaning of their rights, they did not comprehend them at the time the waiver was made. A detailed inquiry is required in these cases. The expert must ask how and when the defendant learned about her rights. Did her lawyer educate her? Did the defendant discuss the rights with other inmates? Did she go to the law library and review case law on this issue? At times, defendants report they have read case law on *Miranda* waivers. Closer questioning, however, may reveal that the law librarian or another inmate located the cases, and provided a verbal summary to the defendant. Asking the defendant to explain the holdings of each case often reveals little or no practical understanding of what she was shown or was explained to her. Explanations are frequently simplistic, described in a rote fashion and inaccurate, revealing a lack of understanding as to the actual holding of the case they have cited. Furthermore, it is not unusual for defendants who claim that they *now* understand their rights, to demonstrate imperfect comprehension when asked to explain them.

Defendant's Reaction to Being Interrogated

Only the defendant can provide the evaluator with information about her reactions to being accused of an offense; separated from friends and family; placed in an interrogation room; and perhaps, surrounded by interrogators who urged her to sign away her Constitutional rights and confess to a crime that she may or may not have committed. Again, it is it unfortunate that this key source of information, the defendant, is the person with the most to gain by presenting an inaccurate or distorted picture of her thoughts and reactions at the time of interrogation. Nonetheless, the information provided by the defendant should serve as data for the expert to consider when formulating an opinion. The information that the defendant provided could generate hypotheses, and the expert should evaluate the likelihood of these hypotheses by examining data gathered during the interview, through testing, through record-review, and from third-party interviews. Such hypotheses might include:

- The defendant was intimidated, overwhelmed, or otherwise did not attend to the rights as they were presented;

- The defendant found it difficult to resist police pressure to waive her rights and confessed to a crime she may or may not have committed;

- The defendant was highly anxious and frightened at the time of interrogation and naively suspended belief; embraced promises or threats made by interrogators, whether real or imagined; and waived her rights, and provided information about her involvement in the crime;

- The defendant hoped that by cooperating with police, she could return home and, thus, signed a document she did not fully understand;

- The defendant felt ignorant about her rights, but she was too embarrassed to admit that she was unable to understand the rights that the police read to her and to appreciate what she was signing;

- The defendant had grown weary of police demands that she waive her rights, rights she understood only imperfectly. She may have signed the waiver with the belief that a lawyer would "sort everything out" sometime in the future;

- The defendant, a former boxer with evidence of brain damage and sub-average intelligence, confessed to a crime he claims he did not commit. He did not fully appreciate his *Miranda* rights, convinced that he should confess to police so that he could later sue the municipality for false arrest and become a millionaire;

- The defendant possesses the cognitive abilities and personality characteristics to fully understand the *Miranda* rights and to resist interrogator coercive strategies (if used) to have made a knowing, intelligent, and voluntary waiver.

Again, all of these scenarios represent *only* hypotheses, generated by the expert, based on information provided by the defendant, to explain why the defendant may not have been able to provide a knowing, intelligent, and valid waiver of rights at the time of interrogation. The expert must thoroughly evaluate any and all hypotheses by examining them within the context of other data obtained, particularly data from independent sources.

Do Miranda-type Warnings Exist in the Defendant's Country of Origin?

The failure of defendants from other countries to adequately comprehend *Miranda* warnings may be partially attributable to the fact that these protections, literally, are foreign to them. That is, such rights do not exist in most other countries, and they may not exist in the defendant's country of origin. The defendant does not understand that suspects are afforded such protections, and she may not even be able to imagine that such protections could exist. A defendant from a small village in India reported that common interrogation practices included hanging suspects by their feet in public places and beating the soles of their feet until they confessed. A call to a former chief of police from a small city in India, now living in the United States, confirmed this practice. As such, a partial explain of why a defendant might lack *Miranda* waiver capacities might lie in the fact that such rights are inconceivable to her, literally and figuratively foreign to her way of thinking and her expectations of how police interrogations are and should be conducted.

Need for an Interpreter in *Miranda* Rights Waiver Cases

If English is the defendant's second language or if the defendant speaks no English, a court-certified interpreter is required. Such individuals are highly trained and recognize the significance that each word they use in their interpretations could have on the outcomes of those cases. They are fully aware that a defendant's responses should not be summarized or in any other way modified—they must be translated verbatim. If a defendant's answer to the forensic mental health expert's question rambles, involves an inappropriate word or concept, or otherwise makes little sense, court-certified interpreters recognize they should not attempt to modify or otherwise "clean up" or make sense of a response that makes little or no sense in the first place. Skilled interpreters frequently make notes during the evaluation, including information to tell the expert at the end of the assessment (e.g., "She makes little sense in her own language;" "She makes up or misuses words that don't exists in her own language;" "She appears to 'tune out' and has problems paying attention"; "Even though her explanation would not make sense in the United States, it is consistent with superstitions that are common in the culture in which she grew up"). These insights may be important for the expert to consider when formulating an opinion.

As discussed in some detail earlier, if the rights were read or shown to the defendant in English, a language in which she has difficulties communicating, the use of an interpreter to interpret the rights into her native language may be inappropriate. The forensic mental health expert is not interested in the capacity of the defendant to comprehend rights in her own language. Rather, the focus of the assessment is on an individual's capacity to understand and appreciate the rights as they were presented to her—most typically in English or Spanish (in which case the use of a certified Spanish-speaking interpreter would be appropriate).

BEST PRACTICE
If a defendant does not speak English, or English is not her first language, a court-certified interpreter is required for the evaluation.

A recent study examined 121 Spanish versions of *Miranda* rights warnings and found that translation errors, from the original English-language version, ranged from minor to substantial (Rogers, Correa, Hazelwood, Shuman, Hoersting, & Blackwood, 2009), with "some Spanish translations [failing] to address the fundamental right to silence or right to counsel" (p. 64). In addition, the Spanish translations appeared to provide less information about *Miranda* rights than did the English versions. As such, the expert may wish to receive feedback from a certified Spanish-speaking interpreter about the adequacy of a Spanish version of the warning, even if it was preestablished, printed, and not translated on the spot. The expert should also inquire about accuracy, regardless of the language into which the warnings were translated.

Defendants from Special Populations

Evaluating defendants from special populations (e.g., youth, mentally retarded, mentally ill, culturally diverse) can present challenges to forensic mental health evaluators. In the sections that follow, we provide some comments about working with defendants who are members of these specialized groups.

EVALUATING JUVENILES

Juveniles tend to have difficulty providing knowing and intelligent waivers of rights, and these difficulties are particularly pronounced

5
chapter

in youth under the age of 15 (e.g., Grisso, 1981; see chapter 3 for a thorough review of the research in this area). Thus, forensic mental health examiners who conduct *Miranda* waiver evaluations will be likely to encounter juvenile defendants. They should, therefore, be familiar with the unique legal and ethical issues associated with conducting evaluations with children and adolescents. They should also be familiar with developmental literature and experienced with age-appropriate methodological approaches.

Regarding the legal and ethical issues associated with evaluating juveniles, the expert must obtain informed consent from the child's legal guardian (parent or court-appointed child advocate) or attorney, unless the assessment was court ordered; the expert should also seek assent from the youth. The expert should explain to the youth the nature and purpose of the evaluation, as well as the limits to confidentiality, in language the child can understand—this requires that the expert have enough experience with youths in this population to grasp both the linguistic and conceptual limitations expected, and to tailor explanations to that youth's level.

Furthermore, the forensic mental health evaluator should be familiar with the broad developmental literature on children's cognitive development and decision making, as well as with the developmentally related, specific literature on juveniles' *Miranda* rights waivers. Familiarity with this literature should help guide the evaluator's questions to include assessment of common conceptual difficulties among juvenile defendants (e.g., failure of many youth to view a right as a privilege—to understand that an adult authority figure cannot revoke a right from a child) (see chapter 3 for a review of common *Miranda* rights misunderstandings among juveniles). In addition, the expert must be familiar with age-appropriate methodological approaches to evaluating a juvenile's capacities to have waived rights. Such an evaluation would require experience with assessment tools designed for youth, experience interpreting juveniles' performance on assessment instruments, and appreciation of

BEST PRACTICE

Obtain informed consent from the juvenile's legal guardian, as well as from the youth himself. Be sure to use language the youth can understand.

the potential validity of a youth's inconsistent performance within and across measures (i.e., youth can acquire more advanced skills and knowledge before they acquire some more basic skills and knowledge). See Otto and Goldstein, 2005, for a description of the process of conducting assessments of juveniles' capacities to have waived *Miranda* rights.

EVALUATING MENTALLY RETARDED DEFENDANTS

Conducting any forensic mental health assessment with defendants classified as mentally retarded brings with it a myriad of potential problems, such as difficulty obtaining informed consent and the inappropriateness of some tests and tools. Furthermore, the defendant may show difficulty understanding the expert's questions and providing focused, relevant, informative answers. She may also have trouble concentrating, maintaining attention, and staying interested in the evaluation, which, under typical circumstance, can require many hours over multiple sessions. The expert must use simple language and clarify the defendant's answers. Parents and other relatives may play even more important roles as providers of third-party information than is typically the case, providing information about the defendant's condition at birth; problems in school and in social functioning; ability to function independently; ability to attend to self-care needs; and ability to understand simple instructions. Certainly, if a parent or other third party was present at the time the rights were administered, the expert should ask about that person's observations of the waiver and interrogation process and should obtain that person's recollections of any advice she gave the defendant. The expert should factor that third-party information into the data that serve as the basis of the expert's opinion. If the defendant has more than one parent or significant third party, the expert should interview each person separately, one immediately after the next (if the parties know one another); between interviews, the expert

BEST PRACTICE
For evaluations of mentally retarded defendants, parents and other relatives may play even more important roles as providers of third-party information than is typically the case. Be sure to interview all significant third-parties (e.g., parents) separately and immediately one after another.

5
chapter

should attempt to limit the communication between these parties to prevent discussion about questions asked and answers given.

EVALUATING INDIVIDUALS WITH SEVERE MENTAL ILLNESS

On occasion, a defendant may present with serious mental illness. The decision to conduct a validity of *Miranda* rights assessment at that time is one that should be decided on a case by case basis. In general, we recommend that if there is no claim or evidence that the defendant was in a seriously mentally ill state when she executed the waiver, the expert should not evaluate the defendant while she is in such a state; such an evaluation could distort the expert's impressions about the defendant's capacities to have waived rights at the time of police questioning. In contrast, records may indicate or the defendant may claim that she was in a floridly symptomatic state of mental illness at the time that she was taken into police custody and rights were read. In such a case, the forensic mental health expert should evaluate the defendant in a similar state, if possible. This approach could produce information that is extremely relevant to the defendant's capacities at the time of the actual waiver. In court, the expert will need to explain to the judge her reasoning behind the decisions she made about how to conduct the evaluation.

EVALUATING THOSE FROM CULTURALLY DIVERSE BACKGROUNDS

When evaluating a defendant from another country, the evaluator should attempt to learn whether a *Miranda* rights equivalent exists in that individual's country of origin. A defendant may have difficulty understanding and appreciating rights if she lacks familiarity with the concept of constitutionally guaranteed protections during police interrogations. In addition, people from some multicultural backgrounds may be very reluctant to reveal information of a personal nature to a stranger or, for that matter, to *anyone* outside of the immediate family.

Traits and abilities of individuals from multicultural backgrounds, whether born in or immigrated to the United States, can be misrepresented by scores on tests commonly used in clinical and forensic psychology. The item content and nature of some tasks may distort interpretation of test results. Such potential for distortion does not necessarily mean that these instruments cannot be given. However, caution should be used in interpreting their results. Given these challenges, the forensic mental health examiner should have experience conducting assessments of people from diverse backgrounds and should consult someone familiar with the defendant's culture if the expert does not have that experience with that culture. Such consultation can help the evaluator develop questions to obtain important information and interpret data when preparing the report and offering testimony.

Collateral Information

Best practice in forensic mental health assessment requires that the expert obtain and rely on corroborative material when collecting data and in formulating opinions. As discussed in chapter 4, the expert should request relevant records from the referring attorney when the referral is accepted, and the expert should conduct collateral interviews with third parties. During the evaluation, the defendant will probably provide information that will point to other possible sources of information to support or refute information provided by the defendant or hypothesized by expert.

When evaluating a juvenile defendant, parents may provide information about the youth's ability to function independently (i.e., free from adult guidance) in a range of settings. Parents may provide observations (which should, of course, be cross-checked against other sources) regarding the child's general comprehension, decision-making abilities, medical and mental health, trust or distrust of others, and need to please and conform. Parents' anecdotal data may help answer questions about whether the youth could knowingly, intelligently, and voluntarily waive *Miranda* rights. Interviews with teachers and the school guidance counselors may provide corroborative information about the juvenile's

5
chapter

cognitive and functional limitations that are relevant to youth's capacities to have executed a valid rights waiver; these parties, typically, are considered to be less biased in their responses, and, therefore, their answers can provide powerful sources of information to guide the expert's opinions. When evaluating adults, third parties (e.g., parents, spouses, former teachers, probation officers, therapists, supervisors at group homes, coworkers) serve similar functions.

Administering Traditional Psychological Tests

When conducting a forensic mental health assessment on the *Miranda* waiver issue, the expert is aware that, ultimately, the judge is interested in the *totality of circumstances* that may have affected the defendant's abilities to have waived *Miranda* rights knowingly, intelligently, and voluntary. In other words, the expert must assess those characteristics of the defendant and/or consider those characteristics of the interrogation that may have interfered with the defendant's abilities to understand the meaning of her rights, appreciate the consequences of waiving those rights, and waive those rights free from unacceptable levels of police coercion. No traditional psychological test has been designed specifically for this purpose, and no traditional psychological test provides information that bears *directly* on these legal competency constructs. Nonetheless, traditional psychological testing may provide data that indirectly assist the expert and the court by explaining *why* a specific defendant may or may not have been capable of making a valid *Miranda* waiver.

If there are questions about the defendant's cognitive abilities—raised during the interview, reflected in the records, or revealed by third parties—the expert should administer an objective measure of intelligence (e.g., Wechsler Intelligence Scale for Children –IV [WISC-IV] or Wechsler Adult Intelligence Scale - IV [WAIS-IV]). It is inappropriate to use an abbreviated measure of intelligence (e.g., Wechsler Abbreviated Scale of Intelligence) in this forensic context. In our opinion, it is not worth the time savings to sacrifice potentially important, objective information on a range of verbal and nonverbal intellectual abilities that may be required to focus on new information, understand that information, apply that information to a specific situation, and make appropriate decisions— all skills required to make a knowing, intelligent, voluntary waiver of *Miranda* rights.

Similarly, if the defendant presents with, or records indicate the possibility of, an underlying neurological dysfunction, neuropsychological testing may be needed. These tests will not reveal whether the defendant has the requisite capacities to waive her *Miranda* rights. However, findings may suggest reasons why she could have had difficulty understanding her rights and applying the rights to silence and counsel to the interrogation situation. If the expert does not have the background, experience, skills, training, or knowledge to administer and interpret neuropsychological tests, an appropriate referral should be made to a board-certified neuropsychologist with experience conducting *Miranda* waiver evaluations.

The expert should administer the Wide Range Achievement Test (WRAT-IV), Wechsler Individual Achievement Test –II (WIAT-II), or other psychometrically sound measure of academic skills if questions have been raised about the defendant's ability to have understood the rights that the police read to her or to have grasped the meaning of the rights printed on the *Miranda* waiver form that she signed. The words included in these instruments are not from the *Miranda* warnings nor included in the *Miranda* rights waiver forms; nonetheless, performance on these tests can help explain why a specific defendant may or may not have had the ability to comprehend her rights.

If questions have been raised about the presence of mental illness, the forensic mental health evaluator should consider administering an objective personality measure, such as the Minnesota Multiphasic Personality Inventory-2 (MMPI-2) or Personality Assessment Inventory (PAI), as well as symptom-specific measures (e.g., ADHD Rating Scale-IV), if relevant. These instruments may help to assess a defendant's current emotional state and may provide insights about the defendant's personality characteristics. Of course, the evaluator is ultimately interested in the defendant's mental state at the time she waived her rights, so present-state information is only helpful insofar as it can facilitate this reconstruction. These data are more objective than judgments based solely on interview data.

Findings from objective personality measures, such as the PAI and MMPI-2, may be particularly relevant when questions have been raised about voluntariness, as required under *Miranda*. Similarly, if assessing factors that might have contributed to a coerced confession or a confession whose trustworthiness is in question, these instruments may provide relevant data. Traits involving submissiveness, conformity and acquiescence, findings of a lack of adequate coping skills or tendencies to be easily threatened, and tendencies toward personality decompensation may be relevant to these issues. Notably, however, all of these instruments require minimum readings levels. As such, their use with defendants with suspected or documented mental retardation, language problems, or reading difficulties would be inappropriate.

Measures of intelligence, academic skills, neurological functioning, personality, and symptom presentation are usually normed on specific populations. Many individuals who are referred for an evaluation of validity of *Miranda* rights waivers are from culturally diverse groups. Yet, with appropriate explanation in the written report and during testimony, data derived from these measures may be of value in corroborating findings that relate to capacities to waive *Miranda* rights.

BEST PRACTICE

You may wish to administer all or some of the following types of measures when conducting a *Miranda* waiver evaluation:

- Measures of intelligence—if there are questions about the defendant's cognitive abilities

- Neuropsychological measures—if there is a possibility of neurological dysfunction

- Measures of academic skills—if the defendant has problems with comprehension

- Objective personality measures—if mental illness is present

Administration of Forensic Assessment Instruments

Grisso (1986, 2003) described a wide range of forensic assessment instruments that have been developed since the early 1970s, including tests, questionnaires, structured interviews, decision-trees, and rating scales. All of these types of instruments can be used to help forensic mental health experts focus their evaluations on the relevant legal criteria underlying the psycholegal referral question. In evaluating the capacities of a defendant to have validly waived *Miranda* rights, Grisso (1998b) developed a set of four instruments—tools that have become part of the standard of practice in assessing this psycholegal issue (DeClue, 2005; Oberlander, Goldstein, & Goldstein, 2003; Melton, Petrila, Poythress, & Slobogin, 2007; Otto & Goldstein, 2005).

Grisso's (1998b) Instruments for Assessing Understanding and Appreciation of Miranda Rights

Overall, courts have admitted testimony based on Grisso's (1998b) *Miranda* instruments, with implicit or explicit acceptance under *Daubert* and *Frye* (e g , *Garner v. Mitchell*, 2007; *United States v. Jackson*, 2006; *Commonwealth v. Woods*, 2004; *People v. Carroll*, 2001; *State v. Caldwell*, 1992). In a few cases (e.g., *Carter v. State*, 1997; *State v. Griffin*, 2005; *People v. Hernandez*, 2007), however, courts have not accepted testimony based on *Miranda* testing. Notably, in these cases, the experts had insufficient experience with the instruments and/or failed to provide complete and accurate testimony about the instruments' admissibility data; the courts' decisions to reject the testimony were not based on the actual characteristics of the instruments but on the inaccurate testimony of the experts who attempted to use those instruments without the proper knowledge, training, or experience with these specialized tools. The few cases that have rejected *Miranda* comprehension testimony underscore the importance of experts understanding and testifying fully about the use, reliability, and validity of the instruments. Fulero (2009) reviewed, in detail, some cases that address the admissibility of these instruments.

See chapter 3 for a detailed description of Grisso's instruments, including descriptions of the instrument development process, the psychometric properties of the instruments, acceptability of the instruments, and the research involving the instruments.

5
chapter

Instruments to Evaluate Voluntary Waiver of Rights

There are no instruments available that directly assess the voluntariness of a rights waiver. Given that case law has established that voluntariness must be based on police behaviors during interrogation (e.g., *Colorado v. Connelly*, 1986), psychological testing of the defendant cannot *directly* address this issue. Nonetheless, psychological testing can provide information about characteristics of the defendant that might have made her more or less susceptible to specific police behaviors. For instance, suspects with mental retardation tend to be highly susceptible to accepting misleading information from authority figures (Everington & Fulero, 1999; Shaw & Budd, 1982), and police may take advantage of this suggestibility by providing information about the offense and strongly encouraging the defendant to take responsibility for that information provided, either through intimidation or implied incentives that the defendant does not have the intelligence to know are untrue. Although, in this example, psychological testing cannot reveal anything about the behavior of the police, the expert should consider administering an instrument to evaluate the suggestibility of the defendant to negative feedback and leading questions from an authority figure during interrogation. The *Gudjonsson Suggestibility Scales* Gudjonsson, 1984, 1987) were developed because "there was a need for such an instrument to assess pre-trial criminal cases involving retracted confessions" (Gudjonsson, 1992, p. 131).

There are two forms of this instrument, GSS1 and GSS2; they can be used interchangeably and have "very similar norms" (Gudjonsson, 1992, p. 133). Gudjonsson reported data on both the reliability and validity of these instruments, and DeClue (2005) indicated that these scales reliably measure "individual differences in interrogative suggestibility. . . . " (p. 160). The defendant is read a brief narrative. She is then asked to recall as much information as she can about the story, both immediately and after approximately 50 minutes. Questions are asked, some of which are subtly misleading. Then, even if the questions are answered correctly, the evaluator informs the defendant that she made a number of errors, must answer the questions again, and should try to be more accurate this second time. Responses are scored to provide information about changes in answers that reflect responses to negative feedback (Shift), susceptibility to leading questions prior to receiving negative feedback (Yield 1) and after receiving negative feedback (Yield 2), and major distortions while recalling the story (Confabulation); a Total Suggestibility score is also provided. Oberlander and colleagues (2003) reported: "The results of this measure, in the context of a multimodal assessment, sometimes provide useful data regarding the existence of suggestibility as a long-term characteristic of the defendant" (p. 353).

Appeal courts have issued conflicting rulings on the admissibility of testimony based upon the GSS. For example, the exclusion of these measures by trial courts was upheld because of a lack of evidence of their scientific validity (*Commonwealth v. Soares*, 2000; *Misskelly v. State*, 1996) and because the concept of suggestibility was not beyond the knowledge of laypersons and would not aid the trier of fact (*People v. Bennett*, 2007). Other courts have upheld the inclusion of findings based upon these instruments (*State v. Romero*, 2003; *United States v. Raposo*, 1998). As such, experts should be aware of any court decisions on the admissibility of data and opinions that arise from the use of the GSS before they decide to use these measures. Fulero (2009) provided a review of a number of these court decisions.

Evaluating Response Style

Most defendants have a clear motive to present themselves as lacking the requisite understanding and appreciation of their *Miranda* rights. Consequently, experts must consider possible malingering or exaggeration; in *Miranda* cases, the expert must evaluate whether the noted deficits are genuine. Here, we suggest a list of ways to assess the critical question of how response style may have shaped a defendant's presentation and answers during interviews, on traditional tests, and on forensic assessment instruments:

- Rely on third-party information and records to corroborate information provided by the defendant;
- Consider the balanced and thoroughness of information provided by the defendant;

- Examine the consistency of the defendant's claimed limitations and her clinical presentation throughout the interviews;

- Administer objective tests of intelligence, memory, and symptoms of mental illness; and

- Administer objective tests that evaluate malingering and exaggeration of cognitive impairment and/or mental illness.

An integral part of any forensic mental health assessment is the use of specialized instruments to assess response style, and "there has been substantial progress in developing and validating these specialized measures during the last seven years" (Heilbrun, Grisso, & Goldstein, 2009, p. 112). If a defendant claims that symptoms of cognitive or mental impairment interfered with her ability to validly waive rights, the evaluator should administer instruments that can assess the validity of these symptoms.

Rogers (2008b) described a number of these measures in detail. Although objective personality tests, such as the MMPI-2 and PAI, contain validity scales to assess response style, the true reading level or cognitive functioning of many defendants referred for *Miranda* waiver evaluations may be too low for these measures. If it is inappropriate to administer those measures, or in addition to those measures, the evaluator should consider using symptom-specific measures of malingering or exaggeration, such as those described by Berry and Schipper (2008) to assess feigned cognitive impairment, those described by Sweet, Condit, and Nelson (2008) to evaluate feigned memory loss, and/or those described by Rogers (2008c) to assess for the false presentation of symptoms of mental illness. Again, decisions to use a specific test must be made on a case by case basis, determined, in part, by the defendant's demographic characteristics and nature of the symptoms reported.

What is "Sufficient" Data upon Which to Base an Opinion?

To form an opinion, there must be sufficient data upon which to base it. For practical and financial reasons, it may not be possible for the

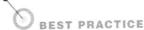

BEST PRACTICE
Consider administering symptom-specific measures to determine whether the defendant is exaggerating or malingering (e.g., feigning cognitive impairment, memory loss, or mental illness).

expert to review all of the records provided or to interview everyone who has knowledge about the defendant at the time the waiver was made. Instead, the expert must only review collateral information until she determines that sufficient information has been gathered to arrive at an opinion. Such a determination can only be made when the expert believes that the information obtained from third-party sources is largely consistent and when additional inquiry becomes redundant. In economic terms, the evaluator has reached the point of diminishing returns, as additional sources are not providing much new information. If there are significant contradictions across data sources, however, the expert must seek additional clarifying information.

There are times when records cannot be obtained: they have been lost, have not arrived in time for the hearing, or are otherwise unavailable. If the information that is lacking is critical to establishing an opinion on the validity of the waiver, the expert should report this to the attorney and ask that the hearing be continued. If, however, a delay will not produce the critical material (e.g., school records were destroyed in a fire), the expert should note in the report and in testimony the absence of those records and how that absence may have affected her opinion.

5
chapter

Conclusions

Experts must collect sufficient data upon which to base an opinion and should rely on multiple sources of information to corroborate findings. The major source of information about the defendant's perceptions of and responses to the interrogation procedure is the defendant. For obvious reasons, information provided by the defendant may

BEST PRACTICE
If critical records cannot be obtained in a timely fashion, alert the attorney and ask for a continuance so that you may request the necessary additional information.

be misleading and should be corroborated by records and third-party sources. The expert should also evaluate the consistency of the information the defendant provides with her behavior during the evaluation. Psychological testing, involving traditional instruments, may help to explain *why* a defendant had problems executing a meaningful rights waiver. Specialized forensic assessment instruments, such as those developed by Grisso (1998b) can also provide objective data specifically about *Miranda* waiver capacities. In addition, experts should consider administering measures specifically designed to assess malingering and exaggeration of symptoms.

Interpretation | 6

After the expert has completed the evaluation of the defendant and collected data from a range of sources, the expert must analyze and interpret all of the information. This chapter focuses on how forensic mental health professionals should approach data interpretation in a manner that is consistent with best practice. How does the expert sift through this data, which can be voluminous at times, to organize it into meaningful, coherent results? How does the expert interpret these results to modify and evaluate hypotheses to form an expert opinion?

A forensic opinion on this or on any psycholegal question is only as good as the data upon which it is based. This chapter assumes that: (a) the expert administered a battery of tests relevant to evaluating the capacity of the defendant to have executed a valid waiver of *Miranda* rights; (b) the administered tests were reliable and valid; (c) tests were scored and rescored to check for errors; (d) during the interviews, the defendant provided sufficient information related to the referral question (e.g., historical data, description of the interrogation, comprehension of the rights administered); and (e) the expert reviewed relevant records and contacted the appropriate third parties.

Consistency of reliable information within and across data sources is the cornerstone of any forensic opinion. That is, in examining and interpreting the data, what consistent patterns or themes emerge that bear directly on the referral question? Ultimately, the report that is to be written and the testimony that may be offered (the topics of chapters 6 and 7) are direct by-products of the interpretative stage of the evaluation process. The credibility of the expert's opinions is based, in part, on the link between the data and the reasoning he used to arrive at his opinions.

The Nature of Hypothesis Testing

Heilbrun (2001) addressed hypothesis testing in his principles of forensic mental health assessment. He emphasizes the importance of verifying information from one source of data if it is to contribute to an expert opinion. He wrote: "Independently obtained information on a second measure about the same construct can be used to support (or refute) hypotheses that may have been generated by the results of the first measure. Thus, impressions from a psychological test in the forensic context should most appropriately be treated as hypotheses subject to verification through other psychological tests, history, medical tests, and third-party observations" (p. 106). The need to evaluate hypotheses by examining information across data sources has been emphasized by many experts in forensic mental health assessment (Goldstein, 2003, 2008; Grisso, 1986, 1998, 2003; Heilbrun, DeMatteo, Marczky, & Goldstein, 2008; Heilbrun, Grisso, & Goldstein, 2009; Kruh & Grisso, 2009; Packer, 2009; Shapiro, 1991; Witt & Conroy, 2009).

Heilbrun (2001) indicated that experts should use scientific reasoning when establishing a connection between the clinical condition of the defendant (as reflected in the data) and the functional psycholegal capacity required by the relevant statues. In the case of *Miranda* waiver evaluation, the expert should focus on the link between the clinical findings and the capacity of the defendant to make a knowing, intelligent, and voluntary waiver of the *Miranda* rights. "When such hypotheses are accepted or rejected according to how well they account for the greatest amount of information with the simplest explanation, the scientific principle of parsimony is applied" (Heilbrun, Grisso, & Goldstein, 2009, p. 113). Heilbrun (2001) explained, "Parsimonious interpretation involves determining which explanation is 'best,' in the sense that it is the least complex while accounting for the most data" (p. 207).

Relevant Hypotheses to Examine

Miranda rights waivers must be made knowingly, intelligently, and voluntarily. The job of the expert at this stage of the evaluation process is to operationalize these legal competency constructs (Grisso, 1986). The data, then, should be examined in light of their relationship to these constructs. In other words, what is the degree of fit between the information collected and these legally required abilities?

Knowing and Intelligent Waiver of Rights

As described in chapter 2, the knowing requirement of a valid waiver is operationalized in psychological terms as "understanding"—to what degree did the defendant understand the basic meaning of rights at the time he waived them and offered the incriminating statement? The intelligent requirement is operationalized as "appreciation"—to what degree could the defendant apply the rights to his own situation and appreciate the consequences of waiving those rights?

When evaluating data for the *knowing* and *intelligent* requirements of a valid *Miranda* waiver, the expert may generate a number of hypotheses. Some examples include:

- The defendant was capable of waiving all of the *Miranda* rights, consistent with the *knowing* and *intelligent* legal requirements;

- The defendant did not understand (in part or in full) one or more of the *Miranda* rights;

- The defendant understood the basic meaning of all of his *Miranda* rights but failed to appreciate the role of the lawyer as an advocate for the suspect;

- The defendant demonstrated evidence of malingering or exaggeration that does not allow the expert to reach an opinion on this issue or which suggests that, in spite of such evidence, the defendant did not understand (in part or in full) one or more of the *Miranda* rights.

- There is insufficient information to offer an opinion about these criteria. As best expressed by Heilbrun (2001), "the parsimonious conclusion is, 'I don't know'" (p. 208).

When considering data related to the *knowing* requirement, the expert should review performance on objective assessment measures that can provide information about the defendant's ability to understand the meaning of information. Such assessment measures include traditional psychological tests (e.g., of intelligence, reading comprehension, listening comprehension), forensic measures of *Miranda* capacities (i.e., the CMR, CMR-R, and CMV of the *Instruments for Assessing Understanding and Appreciation of Rights*), and tests evaluating malingering or exaggeration of symptoms. The expert should also evaluate performance on any standardized tests (e.g., reading comprehension) that were administered to the defendant while in school to compare the consistency of performance on similar abilities across time. In addition, the expert should consider his observations about the defendant's ability to understand his questions and information provided during the interview. These sources of information should be supplemented by any other data the expert has collected that may provide information about the defendant's capacities to have heard, understood, and/or read the words contained in the *Miranda* warnings and to have grasped the overall meaning of each *Miranda* warning statement at the time he waived his rights.

When considering data related to the *intelligent* requirement, the expert should review performance on objective assessment measures that can provide information about the defendant's ability to appreciate his rights—to consider each right, apply it to the interrogation situation, weigh the pros and cons of invoking or waiving the right, and make a reasoned waiver decision based on this comprehension. It is important to recognize that defendants are legally permitted to make decisions that are not in their best interests, provided that they were able to comprehend the relevant information and think through the decision, unimpaired by cognitive impairment or emotional disturbance. The forensic mental health evaluator should consider a range of data sources, including traditional psychological tests (e.g., of intelligence), forensic measures of *Miranda* capacities (i.e., the FRI of the *Instruments for Assessing Understanding and Appreciation of Rights*), observations about the defendant's comprehension of the informed consent process, interviews with third parties about the defendant's reasoning abilities, and any other data related to the defendant's abilities to appreciate the significance of *Miranda* rights and the consequences of waiving them.

There is a related question that must be considered when interpreting data addressing *Miranda*'s knowing and intelligent requirements. How much comprehension is required for a waiver to be meaningfully made? That is, must *all* of the *Miranda* rights be fully understood? What if the defendant understands three of four rights but his comprehension of the fourth right is completely or partially lacking? What if the defendant has an imperfect understanding of some or all of the rights, but he possesses some grasp of each of them (i.e., he understands the rights but does not appreciate them)? Typically, each state has its own statute(s) or case law addressing these questions; experts should recognize that the questions about requisite quantity and quality of comprehension must be legally determined by the judge, the trier of fact. For example, in New York, a mentally retarded and neurologically impaired suspect was given his *Miranda* rights prior to questioning. The rights were also paraphrased and explained by the detective. The defendant waived his rights and, ultimately, was convicted. He appealed, claiming that he had not understood his rights. The appeals court (*People v. Williams*, 1984) ruled, "an effective waver of *Miranda* rights may be made by an accused of subnormal intelligence so long as it is established that he or she understood the

CASE LAW

*People v.
Williams* (1984)

● The appellate court
ruled that individuals of
low intelligence are
capable of waiving
Miranda rights so long
as they understand the
immediate meaning of
the warning.

immediate meaning of the warnings." Furthermore, the court opined, "an inability to comprehend the import of the *Miranda* warnings in the larger context of criminal law generally does not itself vitiate the validity of the waiver." As such, according to this case, "The defendant does not need to understand the advantages of remaining silent, or how statements can be used in court, or the advantages of having an attorney." In another New York case, a defendant claimed that intellectual limitations interfered with her ability to execute a valid *Miranda* waiver (*People v. Marx*, 2003). The appellate court held that her mental retardation did not rise to a level "so great as to render the accused *completely incapable* of understanding the meaning and effect of [the] confession [emphasis added]." The court indicated that "The inquiry focuses on [the] defendant's ability 'to grasp the basic concepts that [she] could refuse to talk to the investigator or that [she] could ask to speak to a lawyer."

Simply stated, in most jurisdictions "defendants must possess only a minimal or concrete understanding of the *Miranda* warnings" (Oberlander, Goldstein, & Goldstein 2003, p. 341). These cases, along with others, suggest that, when considering data on the *quality* of the defendant's *Miranda* rights comprehension, the expert's role is not to testify about whether comprehension of rights was sufficient to validate or invalidate a waiver. Instead, when interpreting data relevant to *Miranda*'s knowing and intelligent requirements, the expert should consider *any* difficulty fulfilling these requirements and

BEWARE
It is not your
role to determine whether
the defendant understood
his rights well enough to
waive them. This is up to the
court to decide.

include this information in the subsequent report. It is, then, up to the court to determine the legal adequacy of the defendant's comprehension of the *Miranda* warnings.

Voluntary Waiver of Rights

As described in chapter 2, the voluntariness requirement of a valid waiver does not have a direct, operationalizable parallel in psychology. Voluntariness must be based on whether police behaviors during the interrogation were coercive (*Colorado v. Connelly*, 1986). This question of coerciveness is, largely, a factual issue for the court to decide, and a forensic mental health evaluator's opinion is not relevant to a judge's decision about whether police behaved in a particular way. Nonetheless, a forensic mental health evaluator can provide information about whether a defendant has characteristics that would have made him particularly susceptible to providing a waiver and incriminating statement, *if* the alleged, coercive police behaviors did, in fact, occur.

When evaluating data for the voluntariness requirement, the expert may generate a number of hypotheses. Some examples include:

- The defendant displayed behaviors or characteristics consistent with the ability to resist alleged police coercion when asked to waive *Miranda* rights;

- The defendant displayed behaviors or characteristics that would increase the likelihood that he would have waived his *Miranda* rights, if placed in the coercive, custodial situation he described; and

- There is insufficient information to form an opinion related to the voluntariness requirement of the waiver.

In many respects, when interpreting data, the issue of voluntariness of the waiver is the most difficult of the three requirements to address. Often, there are major inconsistencies between what the defendant reported happened during the interrogation and what the interrogators said took place. Even if an interrogation was recorded, that memorization may be incomplete—the interaction between the defendant and interrogators may have begun before police initiated the recording. It is a legal, not a forensic mental health, question whether police behavior designed to elicit a confession is acceptable or unacceptable. Often times, the data related to this legal question are absent, insufficient, or unreliable; thus, the expert may not be able to generate an informed opinion. In such a case, only the final hypothesis listed above may be appropriate.

The expert should consider a range of data sources when focusing on the *voluntariness* requirement. If tapes or transcripts of the interrogation exist, the evaluator should carefully review them for any suggestion of factors (situational or related to the defendant's or interrogator's behaviors or actions) that might have increased or decreased the likelihood of an involuntary waiver (e.g., suggestions, promises, manipulation aimed at perceived weaknesses of the defendant, defendant's naïveté or gullibility). The defendant and interrogators' descriptions of the interrogation should be compared with the recording; despite the value in this comparison, the evaluator should recall that the interrogation probably began before taping commenced. The forensic mental health evaluator should review the defendant's personal history, provided by the defendant and third parties. The expert should focus on prior situations in which the defendant may have acquiesced, conformed, or acted in a way that was not in his best interests because of perceived or genuine pressure or manipulation. Observations of the defendant during the assessment session may also be informative on this issue. For example, did the defendant demonstrate an unusual "need to please," a strong need to look to the expert for support or guidance, or a marked tendency to adopt suggestions inadvertently (or purposefully) made by the examiner? If a measure of suggestibility was administered, such as the *Gudjonsson Suggestibility Scales* (Gudjonsson, 1997), are the results consistent with other data? If the defendant possessed the requisite reading level for objective personality testing, it may be particularly relevant to examine his performance on scales that measure personality traits associated with suggestibility, conformity, or difficulty coping with stress.

Addressing Contradictory Data

It is unlikely that every piece of data collected will clearly support or contradict each hypothesis. If the expert were to require consistency among all data, the expert would rarely be able to offer an opinion. More typically, some information provided by the defendant during interviews, reflected in test performance, contained in the records, or provided during third-party interviews will be inconsistent with the vast majority of data obtained on a given topic. In such cases, the expert should carefully examine all of the available, relevant information in order to gauge its accuracy and identify larger trends. Following this careful review, the expert may determine that the atypical information is insufficient to meaningfully contradict these larger trends. Thus, the expert can accept or reject a hypothesis based on most of the information obtained, and offer an informed opinion based on the overall trends. Of course, the expert should be prepared to explain in the report and in testimony why the contradictory information was treated as insufficient to yield a conclusion in its direction.

For example, a hospital record may contain a note indicating that "malingering should be strongly considered." However, no other records or third parties express or reflect this caution, other than to repeat what the original sources indicated. In addition, the expert observes no signs of malingering during the interviews or testing. Consequently, the forensic mental health expert may feel confident about rejecting the hypothesis that the defendant is malingering

BEWARE ⚠
Make sure you are always prepared to explain (in your report and testimony) why you did not take into account any contradictory data.

and embracing an alternative hypothesis that is consistent with the rest of the data.

Misuses of the Available Data

Evaluations of a defendant's capacities to have meaningfully waived *Miranda* rights are retrospective in nature. Data must be examined in terms of the defendant's cognitive and emotional limitations *at the time of the waiver*, free from "contamination" from sources

6
chapter

such as educative intervention or the effects of psychotropic medication. Is the defendant's claim of impaired comprehension at the time of the waiver consistent with the level of functioning at that time, as reflected by multiple data sources? Does the defendant currently possess better comprehension of rights than he claims that he did at the time of the waiver? If so, what may explain this improvement? Or, despite educative interference, does his comprehension of rights remain impaired? In interpreting the data, the expert must be confident that there is sufficient, reliable information to allow him to distinguish between prior and current comprehension. The failure to make this distinction would represent a significant misinterpretation of the data. Lacking such sufficient information, no opinions can be offered.

When assessing the voluntariness of the waiver, the expert would seriously misuse the data if he were to accept at face value the defendant's rendition of what occurred during the interrogation. Similarly, it would be a misuse of the data to accept as fact either the interrogating officer's rendition of events or the recorded evidence; the officers have vested interests in their appearance, and recordings rarely commence at the point of first contact between the defendant and police. Physical or psychological coercion could have occurred prior to the recording or off camera. Thus, when interpreting the data, statements describing the custodial environment must always be viewed as hypotheses. The expert should apply the clinical findings to the issue of voluntariness in an "if/then" paradigm. For instance, *if* such interrogator behavior (e.g., threats) occurred, *then* it is likely, given the clinical findings (e.g., mental retardation and high levels of suggestibility), that the defendant responded in such a manner (e.g., by complying with authority figures' demands). Extreme caution must be taken when examining hypotheses related to voluntariness, and interpretations must be conditional, expressed in terms of conditions that *may* have occurred in the past, unverifiable to anyone, including the expert.

BEWARE
Do not take either the defendant's or the interrogating officer's version of events as fact. Treat all statements as hypotheses to avoid a misuse of data.

Impairments Related to Capacity to Waive *Miranda* Rights

Unlike with criminal forensic mental health evaluations of trial competence (Zapf & Roesch, 2009) or insanity (Packer, 2009), the expert in a *Miranda* waiver challenge case is not required to establish the presence of a mental disease or defect to arrive at an opinion that the defendant did not fully comprehend his rights or have the capacity to withstand coercive police behaviors, if they occurred. Judges may consider virtually any factor under the *totality of circumstances* approach to decide whether rights were validly waived, and they need not base their determination on a specific set of factors (*Fare v. Michael C.*, 1979). Nonetheless, if an expert can identify the reasons why a defendant may have had difficulty executing a valid waiver (e.g., mental illness, mental retardation, neurological impairment), it can improve the utility and credibility of the opinion. Consequently, the expert must review the multiple data sources (e.g., psychological testing, interview, collateral contacts, records) for consistency, and consider the possibility of diagnoses or conditions that may have prevented adequate understanding or appreciating of rights or increased susceptibility to coercive police behaviors, if they existed.

When Can Hypotheses be Accepted or Rejected?

After reviewing the data, the expert must consider each hypothesis to determine its status: should it be rejected or should it become a forensic, psycholegal opinion? As will be discussed in greater detail in chapter 7, when experts testify, they are typically asked about the degree of certainty of their opinions. A common question asked of experts is whether they have reached an opinion to "a reasonable degree of psychological [or psychiatric] certainty." Surprisingly, a thorough review of the legal literature and case law revealed the lack of a precise legal definition of this important construct (Heilbrun, Grisso, & Goldstein, 2009). For example, an Illinois appellate court that attempted to address this issue concluded that there is "no magic to the phrase itself. The phrase provides legal perspective to medical testimony and signals to the jury that a medical opinion is not based on mere guess or speculation"

(*Hahn v. Union Pacific Railroad*, 2004). Lacking legal guidance, what is the level of certainty that forensic mental health experts should have before accepting an hypothesis and adopting it as an opinion? To address this fundamental question, Heilbrun, Grisso, and Goldstein (2009, p. 55) proposed the following threshold:

> Opinions should be data based, including thorough consideration given to all sources of information: comprehensive notes of litigant's interview responses; results of all psychological tests and instruments; information provided by third parties; and a review of records. Relevant studies, published in peer review journals on issues related to the specific case, should be considered as well. Findings should be examined for consistency within and between data sources; major inconsistencies may preclude forming an opinion. Whenever possible, opinions should incorporate sources with established reliability, and with validity for purposes consistent with the present evaluation. Alternative opinions conflicting with the opinions reached, should be considered, and rejected when they are less consistent with all of the information available to the expert.

Heilbrun and colleagues (2009) noted that the use of "such a standard, and providing it to explain one's methodology when asked, is well within the spirit of [Forensic Mental Health Assessment] best practice" (p. 55). Thus, when interpreting the data related to the capacity of a defendant to have executed a valid *Miranda* rights waiver, the expert should accept or reject a hypothesis based on the degree of support provided by an objective examination of the data. If the expert believes that a hypothesis can be supported by citing the consistency of specific data across information sources, then an opinion has been reached. The corollary is true, as well; if the expert can explain that a hypothesis has been rejected based upon the consistency of data across sources, then an opinion has been reached. While this guideline for accepting and rejecting hypotheses is not a substitute for the elusive "reasonable degree of psychological [or psychiatric] certainty" standard, it serves as a model by which hypotheses can be accepted or rejected and adopted as opinions. As a caution, expert witnesses should consider how they would answer the following question asked during cross-examination: "Doctor, you stated you formed an opinion to a reasonable degree of psychological certainty. What do you mean by that term?"

Conclusions

After data have been collected, they must be analyzed and interpreted. The expert needs to examine all of this information for its reliability and consistency across sources. Because the defendant must have waived his rights knowingly, intelligently, and voluntarily, the expert must review the data to determine the degree to which each piece of information is consistent or inconsistent with these requisite abilities. Hypotheses are generated and either accepted or rejected and adopted as an opinion, based upon the determined level of objective, consistent support.

Report Writing and Testimony | 7

A s noted in chapter 1, although this book is comprised of seven chapters, they should not be viewed as covering distinct topics or procedures for conducting an assessment related to *Miranda* waiver validity. Earlier stages of the assessment process are integrated into the later stages and establish the groundwork for the opinions presented in the report and in testimony, if required. In this chapter, we describe the purpose and process of preparing the written report and offering testimony during a suppression hearing.

The Written Report

When to Write a Report

If appointed by the court, the evaluator must usually provide a written report. The expert typically submits a report to the judge, regardless of the findings. The information collected and opinions formed are *not* considered to be attorney-client work product, and the expert has little or no discretion as to whether a report is to be submitted. The judge will make the report available to both the defense and prosecuting attorneys.

In contrast, if the expert has been independently retained by defense counsel, the data collected and opinions reached remain work product, protected by the laws of attorney-client privilege, until the attorney requests that the expert write a report. If no request is made, no report is written. In some jurisdictions, the report may be written but the retaining attorney still has the option of not submitting it into evidence. Generally, the attorney asks for a written report when she believes that, overall, the report

INFO

If appointed by the court, you are required to submit a written report to the judge who will make the report available to both the prosecution and the defense. If retained by the defense, you may or may not be asked to provide a written report.

will be of value to her client in a suppression hearing. Notably, the expert is ethically bound to report *all* relevant data—whether helpful to the client or not—if a report is requested, so the defense attorney's judgment about the expert's findings must be based on the overall information obtained and opinions formed, not on selected information.

For the most part, a prosecutor only requests a *Miranda* evaluation when a defense-referred expert has already reached an opinion suggesting that the defendant may not have had the requisite capacities to provide a valid rights waiver. In such a case, the prosecution-referred expert, typically, will be required to prepare an objective report and may be called as a rebuttal witness. In this situation, the expert will be expected to produce a report, regardless of the findings.

Later in this chapter, we will review procedures for cases in which the expert was asked *not* to prepare a report but, nonetheless, will be asked to testify.

Purposes of a Report in *Miranda* Waiver Validity Cases

Reports on this psycholegal issue serve a number of purposes. The primary purpose is to provide information in written form about the defendant's capacities to have provided a valid waiver of her *Miranda* rights. The role of the expert in these cases is to educate the trier of fact, and the report is a vehicle for doing so. As noted earlier, the defense attorney requests a report if she believes that the information contained in the report will be of value to the client during the suppression hearing, persuading the judge to rule in the client's favor. The lawyer may also believe that a report will be useful when negotiating the plea and sentence; the possibility of having the confession excluded as evidence may influence the prosecutor to propose a more favorable offer to the defense. Occasionally this is why the defense attorney requests a report, but the reason for the request should not affect the expert's opinion. Such opinions should always be data-driven, influenced only by the information relevant to the defendant's capacities to have waived rights. Forensic mental health practitioners should form unbiased opinions directly relevant to psycholegal issues and should not be involved in helping an attorney get a better deal for her client.

In addition to presenting relevant findings to the court, a report on the capacities of a defendant to have executed a valid *Miranda* waiver serves a number of other purposes:

- It helps the expert organize massive amounts of data into a logical, focused summary;
- It helps structure direct examination and helps the attorneys on both sides prepare for expert testimony;
- During direct- and cross-examination, it serves as a "prompt" or outline for the expert, to remind her of the methods used in the evaluation, information obtained through corroborative sources and from the defendant during the interviews and on tests, as well as the nature of the opinions and their underlying reasoning;
- It provides a document that the judge can review in chambers, after testimony has ended, when trying to reach a decision; and
- It may fulfill some jurisdictions' requirements for a work product (e.g., federal cases usually require a proffer, or summary, of the opinions formed and what will be included in the expert's testimony).

Organizing the Report

When determining the structure and format of the report, one size does *not* fit all. There are *many* ways to write a report that conform to best practice standards—and many ways to write a report that fail to meet this threshold. As with all psycholegal evaluations, the expert should structure a *Miranda* waiver report into sections based on the nature of the case and the expert's preference. Of course, the final report must be consistent with ethics standards and with the standard of practice (e.g., all relevant data obtained must be included in the report, not just data that are consistent with the expert's opinion). In terms of the *content* of the report, we describe some general principles here.

GENERAL PRINCIPLES

Reports should reflect both the ethics of the profession (see chapter 4 for a discussion of key ethical issues in this psycholegal area) and the field's accepted practice guidelines (for a review of guidelines, see Goldstein, 2003; Grisso, 1986, 2003; Heilbrun, 2001; Heilbrun, Grisso, & Goldstein, 2009; Heilbrun, Marczyk, & DeMatteo, 2002; Melton, Petrila, Poythress, & Slobogin, 2007; Shapiro, 1991). Key principles an expert should follow in report writing include (but are not limited to):

- Balance and objectivity—include all relevant information, whether positive or negative;

- Thoroughness—include data sufficient to support the opinions reached;

- Relevance—report only information germane to the psycholegal issue;

- Language—use words and concepts comprehensible to non–mental health professionals; the information should not be falsely simplified, but the attorneys and judge should be able to easily understand the material in the report

- Note limitations—describe the limitations of the data

Elements of a Report on Capacity to Have Waived *Miranda* Rights

How the expert chooses to organize the report, in terms of it structure and subheadings, is a matter of individual preference and partly a function of the features of the specific case. Nonetheless, there are some sections or subheadings that are part of the standard of practice in this area and should be included in all reports. (See Heilbrun et al.(2002) for sample reports, on a range of psycholegal topics that are considered to be consistent with best practices.)

Heilbrun (2001) recommends that experts should "Write reports in sections . . . in a way that facilitates the application of various principles [of forensic mental health assessment]" (p. 13). In addition, we believe that the suggested format, tailored, as needed, to the individual facts of a case, helps structure direct examination and helps lawyers prepare for cross-examination of the expert. In addition, use of the suggested format can add credibility to the opinions for two reasons: (1) it can provide a guide to help the expert generate a report directly based on the data, and (2) it provides the expert with the opportunity to testify that her approach to the assessment, report preparation, and testimony was consistent with best practices in the field.

When writing reports addressing a defendant's capacities to have executed a valid waiver of her *Miranda* rights, the expert might consider using the following organizational structure:

1. List relevant historical information: defendant's name, date of birth and age; dates interviewed; and date of report.

2. Indicate the referral source and specific reason for the referral (i.e., Why did the attorney have concerns about her client's capacity to execute a valid *Miranda* waiver?).

3. List the multiple sources of information relied upon: the number and length of interviews conducted; location of interviews; tests and forensic assessment instruments administered, noting whether they were independently scored and/or computer-interpreted; records reviewed; names and dates of all third-party interviews and each party's relationship to the defendant; tapes and transcripts of the waiver and confession; research publications reviewed and relied upon to form opinions.

4. Identify any *relevant* information that was not reviewed (e.g., records, third-party interviews), and

explain why it was not reviewed and what impact that may have on the opinions formed.

5. Briefly summarize relevant records, such as:

- *School records* that provided information about scores on objective tests; placement in special education programs, including the reasons for placement (e.g., ADHD, Learning Disability, Mental Retardation, Emotional Disturbance, Behavior Problems); information derived from Individualized Educational Programs (IEPs); retention in a grade or grades; teachers' and counselors' observations and impressions; and evaluations by school psychologists.

- *Medical and hospital records* that provided information about diagnoses and symptoms associated with neurological dysfunction; a documented history of head injury; trauma noted at birth; pediatric records related to suspicions or a diagnosis of ADHD or learning disorder; history of hospitalization; history of drug or alcohol treatment; history of blackouts; history of noncompliance with a medical regimen for conditions that might result in mental confusion, such as psychosis, hemodialysis, or diabetes; inpatient or outpatient treatment for a mental illness; history of reported symptoms, such as delusions, poor judgment, cognitive impairments, inattention, or self-defeating behaviors.

- *Vocational records* that identified job titles, job descriptions, and job responsibilities; length of employment at each site and reasons for leaving; written evaluations and comments from supervisors; and information about who completed the original employment applications and forms, such as those required for health insurance.

- *Military records,* for those who have been the armed services, might have included such relevant information as rank achieved, reasons for a break in rank, type of discharge, disciplinary actions and descriptions of incidents or behaviors that prompted the actions (e.g., confrontation with an authority figure, drug or alcohol abuse), head injury, exposure to life threatening situations or traumatic event, or presence of a service-related disability.

- *Social Security records,* if the defendant applied for and received Social Security Disability payments, that included the date of the application, supporting documents (e.g., evaluations from treating physicians or mental health professionals), and the nature of the identified disability.

- *Group home and assisted living facilities records* that provided information about the defendant's independent functioning, situations requiring supervision, whether a legal guardian was appointed, relationships with peers and caretakers, and judgment and decision-making in an environment in which the defendant a closely observed.

6. Briefly summarize third-party interviews, focusing on information related to possible impairments in the defendant's capacities to have executed a meaningful *Miranda* rights waiver. Such interviews may have been conducted with:

   - *Parents or guardians* who supported or contradicted the history given by the defendant; this is especially important if the defendant is a juvenile. Particular attention in the report should be given to information about early awareness of a "problem": special education history; speech, motor, and cognitive milestones; self-care; ability to function independently (e.g., cook, bathe without reminders, travel independently, manage money); what parents report interrogators told them; whether parents report that they gave permission for police to talk with their child; and what advice, if any, parents say they gave to their child before or during the interrogation.

- *Teachers, school administrators, and guidance counselors* who verify or refute what was told to the expert by the defendant about her academic performance, school difficulties, and need for special educational services. These third-parties may have answered the following important questions: How does/did the defendant function in school? Can she read and understand what has been read? Can she keep up with the rest of the class? If not, what are her problems? Does she have difficulties following instructions or functioning independently?

For adults, in addition to the aforementioned parties, significant others/spouses (legal or common-law), work supervisors, therapists, and/or group home staff may provide relevant information. For juveniles, interviews with therapists and group home staff might be of potential value as well. Often, these parties can report on the defendant's abilities to function independently, make reasoned decisions, manage money, follow directions, and meaningfully understand things that happen to them and around them.

Most of the report focuses on the actual evaluation of the defendant, including only information relevant to the capacities of the defendant to have meaningfully waived *Miranda* rights. Such information would include:

- *Process of obtaining informed consent*: Highly relevant to the referral question are details about what the expert told the defendant, whether there was any need for the expert to repeat and simplify the information, and the degree to which the defendant was able to comprehend the information.

- *History and background*: A summary of relevant details from the defendant's reported history should be included in the report. These might include parental disciplinary methods, school performance and related academic difficulties, medical problems (including head injury and loss of consciousness), conditions requiring long-term medication and side effects of that medication, use of alcohol and drugs, emotional difficulties and any treatment received, employment history (e.g., completing of job applications, job title, responsibilities, reasons for changing jobs), whether she has a driver's license, leisure time activities (e.g., hobbies, newspapers and books read, favorite television programs, movies attended), time spent with friends (e.g., their age, shared activities), and relationships with significant others. In addition, a review of prior charges (juvenile and adult) and previous experience with the police may have provided data about the defendant's perceptions of the police, whether the defendant waived rights during interrogations for prior offenses, and the reasons behind those waiver decisions.

- *Results of testing*: The purpose of each test should be briefly explained. The expert should include a description of the findings of each test that are relevant to the assessment of those functional abilities required to make a knowing, intelligent, and voluntary waiver of *Miranda* rights. For example, performance on the WAIS-IV or WISC-IV should focus on those subtests that tap abilities needed to comprehend the meaning of the *Miranda* waiver. How did the defendant perform on the Information,

Vocabulary, Similarities, and Comprehension
subtests, parts of the WAIS-IV that draw upon
cognitive abilities involving self-expression, and
comprehension, reasoning, and thinking in other
than a highly concrete fashion? How did the
defendant perform on Arithmetic, Digit Span,
and Letter/Number Sequence, measures that
require attention span and concentration? On a
test such as the WRAT-4 or WIAT-II, at what
grade level does the defendant read words? What
is the defendant's sentence comprehension?
Regarding specific comprehension of the
Miranda warnings, how did the defendant
perform on the "Instruments for Assessing
Understanding and Appreciation of *Miranda*
Rights?" Did she demonstrate difficulty
comprehending the same right or rights across
the four instruments tests that comprise this
forensic assessment tool? What were the
"misunderstandings" or the nature of her
inadequate or questionable comprehension? How
do the defendant's scores compare to those of
the normative samples, and how consistent are
her scores with others of her age and measured
level of intelligence? How did the defendant's
performance on these instruments compare with
her spontaneous recall and understanding of the
Miranda rights and with her ability to explain
the rights she was actually administered? If
objective personality testing was administered,
what do the validity scales indicate about the
defendant's response style? Did scores on these
scales affect the interpretation of her
performance on other tests administered? On
tests of malingering, were there signs of
exaggeration or fabrication, and how did
performance on these measures affect

interpretation of other assessment tools administered? If there are questions about the voluntariness of the *Miranda* waiver, how did the defendant perform on scales that evaluate such characteristics as obedience to authority, suggestibility, and conformity?

- *Behavioral observations*: The expert should describe her observations of the defendant's behavior throughout the evaluation. Such observations might include symptoms of an emotional disturbance; sub-average intellectual functioning; and other signs of cognitive, emotional, or volitional problems that might have affected her ability to have executed a valid *Miranda* rights waiver. The expert should note any problems the defendant seemed to have understanding questions, following test instructions, concentrating, thinking logically and rationally, making decisions, exhibiting judgment, or functioning independently. It can help illustrate the problems observed if the author cites examples, using verbatim quotes from the defendant whenever possible.

7. Typically, the final section of the report describes the expert's opinion. If the forensic mental health expert has followed the outline and completed the steps recommended in this chapter and throughout the book, the opinions should be obvious to the reader by the time she reaches this section—and should clearly reflect the information provided in the earlier sections of the report.

STATING OPINIONS
The expert should begin this section by reiterating the basis of the opinions that will follow. For instance, the expert might write: "The following opinions are based upon two interview sessions conducted with the defendant, her performance on the tests and

instruments administered, a review of relevant records, interviews with other individuals, and consideration of relevant research published in the peer reviewed literature." The expert might add, "Each opinion is offered to a reasonable degree of psychological [or psychiatric] certainty," being prepared to describe the process by which data were obtained and interpreted, and conclusions reached.

Opinions should be concise. The language used should be precise and thoughtful, leaving little room for distortion or ambiguity during cross-examination. Examples of such an opinion might include the following statements: "In my opinion, the defendant's understanding of her right to remain silent is incomplete or imperfect," or "The defendant appears to have a number of personality characteristics that, during a stressful interrogation, would have increased the likelihood that she felt threatened during an interrogation, and responded to a perceived threat (whether real or imagined) by acquiescing to the demands of an interrogator, if they were made."

Each opinion should be followed by a brief description of the data that generated this opinion, summarizing the material included earlier in the report. For instance, the expert might write: "As described previously, performance on the WAIS-IV and WRAT-4 revealed problems with reasoning, judgment, attention span, and word reading that would impair the defendant's abilities to fully comprehend her *Miranda* rights. In addition, responses on instruments that objectively assess understanding and appreciation of these rights reflected similar impairments."

The expert should explain the specific ways in which the defendant misunderstood or failed to grasp the significance of each *Miranda* right. For instance, the expert might write: "The defendant explained that the right to remain silent means, 'I can't talk to the police until they tell me I can talk. You have to be polite; my parents always tell me that,'" or, "When asked about the role of a lawyer, the defendant said, 'The lawyer works for the judge.

BEST PRACTICE
The statement of opinion should be concise and followed by a brief description of the data that generated the opinion.

She helps me if I'm innocent, and she helps the judge figure out my punishment if I'm guilty.'"

ULTIMATE OPINIONS

It is our view that experts should not include ultimate issue opinions in their reports or testimony, a view held by a number in the professional literature (Grisso, 1986, 2003; Grisso, Heilbrun, 2001; Heilbrun et al., 2009; Heilbrun et al., 2002; Kruh & Grisso, 2009; Lipsitt, 2007; Melton et al., 2007; Redding, Floyd, & Hawk, 2001; Weissman & DeBow, 2003). Slobogin (1989) indicates that "most commentators, a good portion of them academics, insist on prohibition against any language in clinical testimony or reports that embraces the ultimate legal question" (p. 259). Nonetheless, other respected authorities have argued that, by excluding ultimate opinions, the trier of fact is deprived of potentially valuable information and that penultimate opinions may confuse the matter (Braswell, 1987; Rogers & Ewing, 1989; Rogers & Shuman, 2005).

Regarding cases involving *Miranda* waiver challenges, we recommend that the forensic mental health expert refrain from offering ultimate issue testimony about the validity of a waiver; instead, the expert should offer information and opinions that will help the judge, the trier of fact, make the legal decision about whether the waiver in question was valid.

It should be emphasized that there is no jury in hearings challenging the validity of *Miranda* rights waivers, and judges are unlikely to "blindly" accept ultimate opinions as facts. The judge is well aware that the expert, no matter what credentials she may possess, does not have the expertise or authority to make a legal decision. Of course, even if the expert refrains from including ultimate issue opinions in the report or in testimony, the judge may explicitly ask the expert for an ultimate opinion. The concluding section of this chapter will address how the expert might handle such a question.

BEWARE You should not offer an opinion on the ultimate legal issue. In *Miranda* waiver hearings, it is for the judge to decide whether the defendant knowingly, intelligently, and voluntarily waived his rights.

Length of Report

Attorneys often prefer brief reports, at times expressing the view that, by providing fewer details, opposing counsel is deprived of the opportunity to prepare a focused cross-examination in advance of direct testimony. Nonetheless, experts should write reports consistent with their personal style and prior reports—the length should be dictated by the facts and complexity of the case. Reports must be balanced, including all data relevant to the validity of the waiver, whether positive or negative for the defendant and whether consistent or inconsistent with the expert's opinion. Reasons for the opinions should be delineated. Sources of information should be identified, and obtained information should be summarized. Even if each of these elements is addressed only briefly, it is difficult to imagine how a report consistent with best practices could be limited to three or four pages. In a complex case, when numerous sources of information are considered, reports may be extensive, totaling 25 pages or more.

Drafts of Reports

Lawyers may ask the expert to submit a "draft" of the report before the "final" report is prepared and submitted. We urge against doing so. The expert should submit *one* report to the lawyer, not a series of edited versions. The report should be the sole work of the expert—it is not a joint collaboration, coauthored or influenced by the retaining attorney. If the expert complies with the request for drafts, opposing counsel could ask for the earlier versions during cross-examination.

In terms of the expert's credibility, we believe that it is far better to openly acknowledge imperfections in the report (e.g., typographical errors, incorrect dates) during testimony than to have to explain why the original report was altered.

Expert Witness Testimony

The report usually serves to organize the testimony that the expert will offer during the *Miranda* waiver hearing. In addition, the expert is likely to be cross-examined on information contained in the report, as well as on data used to produce the report. Such data may include interview notes and summaries of corroborative sources of information (all discoverable, if the expert testifies). As such, the expert should be very familiar with the report and the data upon which it was based. Much of what we wrote earlier in this chapter about the organization and content of the report also applies to the expert's testimony. In this section, we will describe how an expert should prepare for testimony. We also will describe how the forensic mental health evaluator should present qualifications as an expert in this specific area of forensic mental health assessment, when on the witness stand. Furthermore, we will review standards of evidence and other issues related to the content of direct and cross-examination testimony (for more detailed information about expert testimony, see Bank & Packer, 2007; Barsky & Gould, 2002; Brodsky, 1991, 1999; Ewing, 2003; Hess, 2006; Lubet, 1998; and Ziskin, 1995, 2000).

Preparing for Testimony

The expert began preparing for testimony upon initially accepting the case. That is, the expert decided that she possessed the expertise required to conduct an assessment of the defendant's capacities to have executed a valid *Miranda* waiver and that she has the background, experience, skills, training, or knowledge required to conduct the evaluation, given the defendant's age, cultural background, and other relevant demographics. The expert should review her curriculum vitae (CV) with the lawyer, and questions appropriate to the forensic mental health profession's expertise evaluating *Miranda* waiver validity should be formulated. (These questions may be asked during voir dire, the process by

BEWARE Be sure that you are very familiar with your report and the data upon which it is based. You are likely to be cross-examined on the information the report contains.

7
chapter

which an individual is examined before being accepted as an expert by the presiding judge).

When selecting tests or instruments, the expert should have considered their reliability, validity, relevance to the psycholegal question, and appropriateness for the specific defendant. The expert will probably be asked questions about each of these issues during testimony.

The expert should review the findings of the assessment with the referring attorney, describing the data upon which the opinions were based. Any questions about the findings that the lawyer might want to ask during direct examination should be reviewed, and the expert's answers should be discussed. The attorney should be sure to review all of the expert's interview notes and record summaries, given that the opposing counsel will probably request a copy of these documents. The expert should thoroughly discuss with the attorney all data and findings that are inconsistent with the final opinions. The attorney and expert should prepare questions that provide the expert with an opportunity to describe these data and findings to the judge. These questions will allow the expert to explain why this information did not substantially affect her opinions. The expert should identify limitations of the opinions and emphasize to the attorney that no questions soliciting ultimate opinion testimony (i.e., whether the defendant could or could not have made a valid *Miranda* waiver) should be asked.

Preparing the Defendant to Hear the Testimony that will be Offered

At times, the expert's findings may be very upsetting, or even traumatic, to the defendant. Her reaction to the testimony may result in increased anxiety, depression, suicidal behavior, or psychotic decompensation. How the defendant reacts during testimony may affect the judge's attitudes toward her—and potentially affect the suppression decision or later sentencing. If the expert believes that the some of the findings may negatively affect the defendant, the expert should review with the defendant the testimony she expects to offer in court. If, after the review, the defendant appears to be "shaken" or to present an increased danger to herself or others, the expert may seek safety precautions, such as informing correctional staff that upsetting information was discussed and a recommendation for close observation.

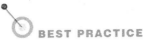

As an example, in one case involving a defendant's capacities to have validly waived his *Miranda* rights, it was discovered during the course of the evaluation that the woman the defendant thought was his biological mother was, in fact, his grandmother. An older brother had raped his sister, and it was she who was the defendant's mother. He had been shielded from this history for obvious reasons. Revealing this information in open court without having adequately prepared the defendant would be unthinkable, creating a range of potential risks during and after the hearing.

Voir Dire or Qualifications

Prior to offering testimony, the judge must determine whether the forensic mental health evaluator qualifies as an expert. Federal courts and most state courts rely on the Federal Rules of Evidence and their respective state equivalents when making this determination. Federal Rules of Evidence (Rule 702) incorporated criteria delineated in *Jenkins v. United States* (1962), which established that an expert is one who possesses "knowledge, skill, experience, training, or education" related to the specific area of testimony. But how does the judge determine whether these requirements are met?

During trial preparation, the expert should have reviewed her CV with the retaining attorney. She should have familiarized the lawyer with those qualifications directly related to the legal standards of expertise that would be relevant in a suppression hearing under *Miranda*. There are no "boilerplate qualifications," no one-size-fits-all list of pro forma questions that the attorney can pull from a file to qualify the expert. Rather, questions must be tailored to the specific psycholegal issue under consideration, the defendant's specific background, and the unique facts of the case. It is

INFO

In qualifying the expert, the court considers

- education,
- training,
- experience,
- credentials, and
- specific work in conducting forensic mental health assessments

useful for the expert to keep a list of qualifying questions relevant to her discipline, position, education, training, professional experience, credentials such as licensure and board certification, and specific work in conducting forensic mental health assessments for the courts on issues such as *Miranda* waiver capacities. This list, which can be supplemented as needed, can be provided to the attorney during preparation.

If the case involves a juvenile defendant, the lawyer should emphasize, in the voir dire examination, the items on the expert's CV that have involved assessing, treating, or conducing research on juveniles. If the expert teaches a relevant course at a university, such as "Psychological Evaluation and Expert Testimony" or "Psychology and the Law," questions should be asked about the content of those courses; specific questions should be asked about what the expert covers in these courses about the laws governing *Miranda* rights waivers and the research and methodology used to conduct these highly specialized assessments. Similarly, the attorney should ask questions about the expert's continuing education teaching, professional presentations, publications, consultation, and supervision of those in training. In each area, the attorney should focus questions on the evaluator's skills, knowledge, experiences, and expertise assessing the defendants in cases evaluating defendants' capacities to waive *Miranda* rights.

What to Bring to Court?

The expert should organize the case-related files so that if asked about a specific document during testimony, she can find it easily. In general, any materials that the expert has relied upon to form an opinion should be brought to court. We also recommend that additional copies of these documents be duplicated in advance, in case the records are to be placed into evidence and that the opposing attorney asks for a set.

BEST PRACTICE
Bring duplicates of all case-related materials to court in case they are to be placed into evidence and/or the prosecution requests copies.

What if No Written Report Was Requested but Testimony Is Required?

If confronted with this scenario, the expert may wish that she were a bit more forceful in convincing the retaining lawyer that a report, however brief, should have been submitted. The expert must now address the court without the benefit of a report on which to rely to refresh memories and to organize testimony. As such, in preparing for court, experts may feel as if they are studying a script for a play, committing essential facts, findings, and opinions to memory. Under the stress of testimony, on which a case may be decided based upon the accuracy and thoroughness of the information presented, there is considerable pressure on the expert. If there is no written report, there is an even greater than usual need to assist the retaining attorney in preparing for direct examination—in a sense, each question, can serve as a prompt for the expert to produce the relevant information that the judge should hear. The lawyer may want to prepare a checklist of important points that the expert needs to cover during testimony, and, if something of significance is omitted, she should ask a question about it.

Observing Testimony of Other Witnesses

It is generally not a good idea for the expert to be present in the courtroom while other witnesses, expert or lay (fact), are testifying. It may give the appearance to the trier of fact that, rather than being an objective party, the expert is an advocate, having an interest in the outcome of the case. Despite this general guideline, however, there may be occasions in *Miranda* hearings when it would be valuable to an expert's findings and opinions if the expert were in the courtroom while another witness testifies. For example, if police interrogators testify about the procedures they used

7
chapter

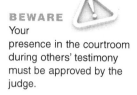

BEWARE
Your
presence in the courtroom
during others' testimony
must be approved by the
judge.

during the interrogation; the length of the interrogation; or the cognitive, emotional, and physical condition of the defendant at the time of interrogation, the expert can incorporate this information into her testimony. In one case, a detective was cross-examined by the defense attorney. After prolonged and probing questioning lasting well over an hour, the detective became irritated by the questions. Spontaneously, and in a resentful tone, he blurted out, "We're not talking about rocket science here. It's only about understanding these simple warnings. It's not as if Donald can't bathe himself or drive a car." In addition to mischaracterizing the rights as "simple," the detective was unaware that the expert had been told by the defendant's parents that two weeks might pass before their son, age 20, would shower (only after encouragement to do so) and that he did not have a driver's license because he was unable to read and understand the learner's permit preparation booklet. At the suggestion of the expert, the defense attorney incorporated questions about the detective's false assumptions into the direct examination of the expert. It is important to note that, in most jurisdictions, the judge must approve a request that a testifying expert be permitted to be present in the courtroom to hear others testify.

Evidentiary Standards

Heilbrun, Grisso, and Goldstein (2009) pointed out that the subject matter of expert testimony is limited by rules of evidence. They explained that, at times, the expert may be required to indicate at an evidentiary hearing, in advance of testimony, the content of the proposed testimony and to provide information about the methodology upon which she relied to form her opinions. "This is more likely if the proposed testimony would address a topic not usually considered by the court (e.g., the likelihood that a defendant has given a false confession) or involves the use of a specialized tool by the expert as part of the FMHA (e.g., instruments related to evaluating the likelihood of sexual violence recidivism)" (Heilbrun, Grisso, & Goldstein, 2009, p. 46). Standards for admissibility of expert testimony exist "to prevent unqualified experts from testifying in the courtroom on the basis of irrelevant or inadequate evidence" (Weissman & DeBow, 2003, p. 47). In the case of proposed expert testimony addressing those factors affecting the validity of a *Miranda* waiver, it is possible that the judge or opposing counsel may question the admissibility of such testimony as it relates to an opinion on voluntariness of a confession or the reliability of instruments used in assessing the knowing and intelligent prong of *Miranda,* such as the "Instruments for Assessing Understanding and Appreciation of *Miranda* Rights."

As Ewing (2003) has emphasized, expert testimony in forensic psychology and psychiatry must have a scientific foundation. Two landmark cases address the criteria by which the admissibility of expert testimony will be decided. *Frye v. United States* (1923) addressed the admissibility of polygraph testimony as a measure of truthfulness. Adopted in all federal and state jurisdictions, and the sole standard of admissibility for sixty years, the *Frye* standard established that expert testimony was admissible if it was "sufficiently established to have gained general acceptance in the particular field in which it belongs" (p. 1014). Later, *Daubert v. Merrell Dow Pharmaceuticals* (1993) was decided. In this case, an experimental study had been conducted to determine if a relationship existed between an antinausea drug and a specific birth defect. The study had been conducted for the purposes of the legal case and testimony based on it was challenged, in part, because it had not been published in peer-reviewed journals or otherwise generally accepted in the scientific community. A broader standard replaced *Frye* on the federal level—whether the testimony would, likely, assist the trier of fact and if the proposed testimony was based on reliable and relevant methodology. Under *Daubert,* judges were given the role of "gatekeeper," using a number of criteria to determine admissibility of testimony. They were to consider whether the technique or theory in question could be tested or was testable, whether it had been subjected to peer review and published, its potential or known error rate, and whether it had been accepted in the scientific community (Heilbrun, Grisso, & Goldstein, 2009). Because *Daubert* was not based on an error of

Frye v. United States (1923)

- The Court held that expert opinion based on a scientific technique is admissible only where the technique is generally accepted as reliable in the relevant scientific community.

Daubert v. Merrell Dow Pharmaceuticals (1993)

- The Court ruled that judges be given the role of "gatekeeper," using a number of criteria (testing, peer review, error rate, and underlying science) to determine admissibility of expert testimony.

- The *Daubert* standard replaced the *Frye* standard at the federal level, but states are free to choose either (or a combination of both) to determine the standard for admissibility of testimony.

Constitutional law, states were left to decide for themselves whether to rely on *Frye* or *Daubert* (or a combination of both) to determine the standard for admissibility of expert testimony.

Experts testifying on issues related to *Miranda* waivers should be aware of the standard used in the jurisdiction in which they will testify. If legal challenges regarding the use of specific instruments or data are anticipated, the expert should have the retaining attorney review case law for prior decisions about their admissibility. The expert should be prepared to address the requirements under *Frye* or *Daubert* if a hearing on admissibility is conducted. The expert should be able to report information about instruments' reliability, validity, use with particular populations, and acceptance in the field. In addition, the expert should be familiar with the peer-reviewed literature on the effects of relevant *totality of circumstances* factors on *Miranda* waiver capacities. It may be important to present this information at an admissibility hearing.

Direct Examination

During direct examination, the retaining attorney will question the expert about the reasons for the referral, the methodology used to evaluate the defendant's capacity to have waived *Miranda* rights, relevant research on the topic, and the opinions formed. Because the expert met with the lawyer and prepared testimony prior to the hearing, the attorney should not be surprised by any of the opinions reached or the data upon which each was based.

As described by Heilbrun, Grisso, and Goldstein (2009), for both direct and cross-examination, the expert should place an emphasis on "the role of teaching, and [on] avoiding the perception of smugness, overconfidence, hostility, or gratuitous humor" (p. 133). Direct examination should be used as an opportunity for the expert to describe data that were inconsistent with the majority of findings or that contradicted the opinions that were generated. For example, records may have indicated that the defendant had a number of prior arrests and, during two previous interrogations, refused to speak with interrogators. If asked how, in spite of this information, the expert could conclude that the defendant did not comprehend the right to remain silent, the expert might explain that the interrogators in those other cases were women, that the suspect was painfully self-conscious and shy around those of the opposite sex (based upon other information), and, in many situations in which women were present in the past, the defendant supposedly became mute (according to third-party sources) The defendant's silence and his agreement that he understood his right to remain silent in prior interrogations may have been related to his general withdrawal when around women—it may not have been an actual decision about his rights, waiver, or decision to participate in the interrogation.

It is important to emphasize that, during direct examination, the expert can provide thorough, detailed answers to questions. This is the opportunity for the expert to clearly and thoughtfully address any concerns the judge might have with her opinions, such as the presence of inconsistent data. If these concerns are not raised during direct examination, opposing counsel might ask about them during cross-examination, using questions that limit the expert's answers to "yes" or "no." Consequently, it is best to address data inconsistent with the expert's opinions during direct examination.

Cross-Examination

Following questioning by the retaining attorney, the expert will undergo cross-examination. Questions are typically designed to weaken the impact of the expert's testimony on the judge's

7
chapter

decision by attacking one or more of the following: the forensic mental health profession, the methodology used, the logic behind the opinions, or the expert's integrity. As is true with any psycholegal testimony, these questions are not personal, and the expert should try not to get flustered or offended. If the expert is familiar with the data; re-scored all of the tests; reviewed the relevant research; presented findings in the report and during direct examination in a balanced, objective, and open fashion; and testified in a manner that upheld the oath to "tell the truth, the whole truth, and nothing but the truth," then cross-examination (although sometimes stressful and uncomfortable) should not be a threatening experience.

Prior to testifying, the expert should anticipate questions that are likely to be asked during cross-examination and prepare answers that are responsive and nondefensive. For example, a common question is, "Couldn't the defendant just be lying when she told you she didn't understand her rights?" The expert can use this question as an opportunity to review the reasons why multiple sources of information were used and to summarize the data that led the expert to reject that alternative hypothesis. During cross-examination, if the expert does not know an answer to a question, a simple "I don't know" is the most honest, effective way to respond. Faking an answer during cross-examination can dig a hold from which the expert may be unable to extricate herself. If the forensic mental health professional is truly an "expert" on evaluating the capacities of a defendant to have executed a valid *Miranda* rights waiver, then she knows more about the topic and related assessment issues than either attorney. This will be helpful in presenting effective and credible expert testimony.

Conclusions

The written report and testimony directly reflect the methods used and data collected during the evaluation. Reports may be required by the judge if the evaluation was court ordered. Otherwise, in most jurisdictions, the expert only writes a report if requested to do so by the referring attorney. A report serves numerous purposes: it organizes the data, summarizes the findings, and presents the opinions and the expert's reasons for forming them. As such, the report structures the content of the testimony that may follow, with the testimony drawing directly on the report. Testimony requires adequate preparation, including meeting(s) with the attorney to review all of the data collected and the opinions reached—including data inconsistent with the expert's opinions. The expert and attorney should discuss questions that will be asked during direct examination, including those about the inconsistent data. The expert should anticipate questions likely to be asked during cross-examination and formulate nondefensive, responsive answers. The expert can take some comfort in knowing that, if she conducted the evaluation thoroughly, consistent with best practices, and wrote the report in a thorough, objective manner, cross-examination will not be as imposing as it might appear.

References

Abramovitch, R., Higgins-Biss, K. L., & Biss, S. R. (1993). Young persons' comprehension of waivers in criminal proceedings. *Canadian Journal of Criminology, 35*(3), 309–322.

Abramovitch, R., Peterson-Badali, M., & Rohan, M. (1995). Young people's understanding and assertion of their rights to silence and legal counsel. *Canadian Journal of Criminology, 37*(1), 1–18.

American Academy of Psychiatry and the Law. (2005). *Ethical guidelines for the practice of forensic psychiatry.* Bloomfield, CT: American Academy of Psychiatry and the Law.

American Medical Association et al. (2003). Brief of the American Medical Association et al. as *amici curiae* in *Roper v. Simmons*. U.S. Briefs 03-633. *Applied Social Psychology, 5*, 147–159.

American Psychiatric Association. (2000). *Diagnostic and Statistical Manual of Mental Disorders* (4th ed., text revision). Washington, DC: American Psychiatric Association.

American Psychiatric Association. (2001). *The principles of medical ethics with annotation especially applicable to psychiatry.* Washington, DC: American Psychiatric Association.

American Psychological Association. (1993). Guidelines for providers of psychological services to ethnic, linguistic, and culturally diverse populations. *American Psychologist, 48*, 45–48.

American Psychological Association. (2002). Ethical principles of psychologists and code of conduct. *American Psychologist, 57*, 1060–1073.

American Psychological Association (2007). Record keeping guidelines. *American Psychologist, 62*, 993–1004.

Appelbaum, P. (1997). A theory of ethics for forensic psychiatry. *Journal of the American Academy of Psychiatry and the Law, 25*, 233–247.

Appelbaum, P., & Gutheil, T. (2007). *Clinical handbook of psychiatry and the law* (4th ed.). Baltimore: Williams & Wilkins.

Archer, R. P., Buffington-Vollum, J.K., Stredny, R.V., & Handel, R. W. (2006). A survey of psychological test use patterns among forensic psychologists. *Journal of Personality Assessment, 87*, 84–94.

Atchison, M., & Keyes, D. (1996). Why Johnny Lee Wilson went to prison. In D. Connery (Ed.), *Convicting the innocent* (pp. 118–126). Cambridge, MA: Brookline Books.

Baird, A. A., Gruber, S. A., Fein, D. A., Maas, L. C., Steingard, R. J., Renshaw, P. F., Cohen, B. M., & Yurgelun-Todd, D. A. (1999). Functional magnetic resonance imaging of facial affect recognition in children and adolescents. *Journal of the American Academy of Child and Adolescent Psychiatry, 38*, 195–199.

Baird, A., & Fugelsang, J. (2004). The emergence of consequential thought: Evidence from neuroscience. *Philosophical Transactions of The Royal Society of London: Series B, 359,* 1797–1804.

Bank, S. C., & Packer, I. K. (2007). Expert witness testimony: Law, ethics and practice. In A. M. Goldstein (Ed.), *Forensic psychology: Emerging topics and expanding roles* (pp. 421–445). Hoboken, NJ: John Wiley & Sons.

Barsky A. E., & Gould, J. W. (2002). *Clinicians in court: A guide to subpoenas, depositions, testifying, and everything else you need to know.* NY: Guilford Press.

Berry, D. T. R., & Schipper, L. J. (2008). Assessment of feigned cognitive impairment using standard neuropsychological tests. In R. Rogers (Ed.), *Clinical assessment of malingering and deception* (3rd ed.) (pp. 237–254). NY: Guilford Press.

Bishaw, A., & Iceland, J. (2003). Poverty: 1999 (Census 2000 brief) (Current Population Reports C2KBR-19). Washington, DC: U.S. Census Bureau.

Blagrove, M. (1996). Effects of length of sleep deprivation on interrogative suggestibility. *Journal of Experimental Psychology: Applied, 2*(1), 48–59.

Blagrove, M., & Akehurst, L. (2000). Effects of sleep loss on confidence-accuracy relationships for reasoning and eyewitness memory. *Journal of Experimental Psychology: Applied, 6,* 59–73.

Blagrove, M., Alexander, C., & Horne, J. A. (1995). The effects of chronic sleep reduction on the performance of cognitive tasks sensitive to sleep deprivation. *Applied Cognitive Psychology, 9*(1), 21–40.

Blagrove, M., Cole-Morgan, D., & Lambe, H. (1994). Interrogative suggestibility: The effects of sleep deprivation and relationship with field dependence. *Applied Cognitive Psychology, 8*(2), 169–179.

Bonovitz, J. C., & Bonovitz, J. S. (1981). Diversion of the mentally ill into the criminal justice system: The police intervention perspective. *International Journal of Psychiatry, 138,* 973–976.

Braswell, A. L. (1987). Resurrection of the ultimate issue rule. *Cornell Law Review, 72,* 620–640.

Brodsky, S. L. (1991). *Testifying in court: Guidelines and maxims for the expert witness.* Washington, DC: American Psychological Association.

Brodsky, S. L. (1999). *The expert expert witness: More maxims and guidelines for testifying in court.* Washington, DC: American Psychological Association.

Cassell, P. G. (1996). *Miranda*'s social costs: An empirical reassessment. *Northwestern University Law Review, 90,* 387–499.

Cassell, P. G., & Hayman, S. B. (1996). Police interrogation in the 1990s: An empirical study of the effects of *Miranda. UCLA Law Review, 43,* 840–931.

Cauffman, E., & Steinberg, L. (2000). (Im)maturity of judgment in adolescence: Why adolescents may be less culpable than adults. *Behavioral Sciences & the Law, 18*(6), 741–760.

Clare, I., & Gudjonsson, G. H. (1991). Recall and understanding of the caution and rights in police detention among persons of average intellectual ability and persons with a mild mental handicap. *Issues in Criminological & Legal Psychology, 1*(17), 34–42.

Cloud, M., Shepherd, G., Barkoff, A., & Shur, J. (2002). Words without meaning: The Constitution, confessions, and mentally retarded suspects. *University of Chicago Law Review, 69,* 495–624.

Colwell, L. H., Cruise, K. R., Guy, L. S., McCoy, W. K., Fernandez, K., & Ross, H. H. (2005). The influence of psychosocial maturity on male juvenile offenders' comprehension and understanding of the *Miranda* warning. *Journal of the American Academy of Psychiatry and the Law, 33*(4), 444–454.

Committee on Ethical Guidelines for Forensic Psychologists. (1991). Specialty guidelines for forensic psychologists. *Law and Human Behavior, 15,* 655–665.

Cooke, D. J., & Philip, L. (1998). Comprehending the Scottish caution: Do offenders understand their right to remain silent? *Legal and Criminological Psychology, 3,* 13–27.

Cooper, V. G., & Zapf, P. A. (2008). Psychiatric patients' comprehension of *Miranda* rights. *Law and Human Behavior, 32,* 390–405.

Covington, M.V., & Omelich, C. L. (1987) "'I Knew It Cold Before the Exam': A Test of the Anxiety-Blockage Hypothesis." *Journal of Educational Psychology* 79:393–400.

Cruise, K. R., Pitchal, E. S., & Weiss, R. (2008). Parental involvement in the interrogation of juveniles: A review of state statutes and implications for research and practice. Presented at the annual conference of the *American Psychology–Law Society*, Jacksonville, FL.

Davies, P. L., & Rose, J. D. (1999). Assessment of cognitive development in adolescents by means of neuropsychological tasks. *Developmental Neuropsychology, 15*(2), 227–248.

Davies, T. Y. (1982). Affirmed: A study of criminal appeals and decision-making norms in a California court of appeal. *American Bar Foundation Research Journal, 7,* 543–648.

DeClue, G. (2005). *Interrogations and disputed confessions: A manual for forensic psychological practice.* Sarasota, FL: Professional Resource Press.

Denkowski, G. C., & Denkowski, K. M. (1985). The mentally retarded offender in the state prison system: Identification, prevalence, adjustment, and rehabilitation. *Criminal Justice and Behavior, 12*(1), 55–70.

Dinges, D. F., & Kribbs, N. B. (1991). Performing while sleepy: Effects of experimentally-induced sleepiness. In T. H. Monk (Ed.), *Sleep, sleepiness and performance* (pp. 97–128). Chichester, U.K.: John Wiley & Sons.

Driver, E. D. (1968). Confessions and the social psychology of coercion. *Harvard Law Review, 82,* 42–61.

Drogin, E. Y. (2009). Therapeutic jurisprudence and jurisprudent science: *Miranda* and mechanisms of legal change. Paper presented at annual meeting of American Psychology–Law Society, Jan Jose, Texas.

Ellis, J., & Luckasson, R. A. (1985). Mentally retarded criminal defendants. *George Washington Law Review, 53,* 414–493.

Evans, J. St. B. T., & Watson, P. C. (1976). Rationalization in a reasoning task. *British Journal of Psychology, 67,* 479–486.

Everington, C., & Fulero, S. M. (1999). Competence to confess: Measuring understanding and suggestibility of defendants with mental retardation. *Mental Retardation, 37,* 212–220.

Ewing, C. P. (2003). Expert testimony: Law and practice. In A. M. Goldstein (Ed.), *Forensic psychology: Vol. 11* of *Handbook of psychology* (pp. 55–680). Hoboken, NJ: John Wiley & Sons.

Federal Rules of Evidence (2001) Washington, DC, U.S. Government Printing Office.

Feeney, F., Dill, F., & Weir, A. (1983). Arrests Without Conviction: How Often They Occur and Why. Washington, DC: U.S. Department of Justice.

Feld, B. C. (2000). Juveniles' waiver of legal rights: Confessions, *Miranda,* and the right to counsel. In T. Grisso & R. G. Schwartz (Eds.), *Youth on trial: A developmental perspective on juvenile justice* (pp. 105–139). Chicago: University of Chicago Press.

Ferguson, A. B., & Douglas, A. C. (1970). A study of juvenile waiver. *San Diego Law Review, 7,* 39–54.

Follette, W. C., Davis, D., & Leo, R. A. (2007). Mental health status and vulnerability to police interrogation tactics. *Criminal Justice, 22,* 42–49.

Fromme, K., Katz, E., & D'Amico, E. (1997). Effects of alcohol intoxication on the perceived consequences of risk taking. *Experimental and Clinical Psychopharmacology, 5,* 14–23.

Frumkin, I. B (2000). Competency to waive *Miranda* rights: Clinical and legal issues. *Mental and Physical Disabilities Law Reporter, 24,* 326–331.

Frumkin, I. B. (2008). Psychological evaluation in *Miranda* waiver and confession cases. In R. L. Denny & J. P. Sullivan (Eds.), *Clinical Neuropsychology in the criminal forensic setting,* (pp. 135–175). New York: The Guilford Press.

Frumkin, I. B. & Garcia, A. (2003). Psychological evaluations and competency to waive *Miranda* rights. *The Champion, 27,*12-23.

Fulero, S. M. (2009) Admissibility of expert testimony based on the Grisso and Gudjonsson Scales in disputed confession cases. *Open Access Journal of Forensic Psychology, 1,* E44-E55 (to appear in the *Journal of Psychiatry and Law,* in press).

Fulero, S. M., & Everington, C. (1995). Assessing competency to waive *Miranda* rights in defendants with mental retardation. *Law & Human Behavior, 19*(5), 533–543.

Fulero, S. M., & Everington, C. (2004). Assessing the capacity of persons with mental retardation to waive Miranda rights: A jurisprudent therapy perspective. *Law and Psychology Review, 28,* 53–69.

Gable, S. L., & Shean, G. D. (2000). Perceived social competence and depression. *Journal of Social and Personal Relationships, 17*(1), 139–150.

Gardner, M. & Steinberg, L. (2005). Peer influence on risk taking, risk preference, and risky decision making in adolescence and adulthood: An experimental study. *Developmental Psychology, 41,* 625–635.

Giedd, J. N., Blumenthal, J., Jefferies, N. O., Castellanos, F. X., Liu, H., Zijdenbos, A., Paus, T., Evans, A. C., & Rapoport, J. L. (1999). Brain development during childhood and adolescence: A longitudinal MRI study. *Nature Neuroscience, 2,* 861–863.

Gogtay, N., Sporn, A., Clasen, L. S., Nugent, T. F., III, Greenstein, D., Nicolson, R., Giedd, J. N., Lenane, M., Gochman, P., Evans, A., Rapoport, J. L. (2004). Comparison of progressive cortical gray matter loss in childhood-onset schizophrenia with that in childhood-onset atypical psychoses. *Archives of General Psychiatry, 61*(1), 17–22.

Gold, J. M., & Harvey, P. D. (1993). Cognitive deficits in schizophrenia. *Psychiatric Clinics of North America, 16*(2), 295–312.

Goldstein, A. M. (2003). Overview of forensic psychology. In A. M. Goldstein, (Ed.), *Forensic psychology: Vol. 11 of Handbook of psychology* (pp. 3–21). Hoboken, NJ: John Wiley & Sons.

Goldstein, A. M. (2008). Forensic psychology: Toward a standard of care. In A. M. Goldstein (ed.), *Forensic psychology: Emerging topics and expanding roles* (pp. 3–44). Hoboken, NJ: John Wiley & Sons.

Goldstein, A. M., Morse, S. J., & Shapiro, D. L. (2003). Evaluation of criminal responsibity. In A. M. Goldstein (Ed.), *Forensic psychology: Vol. 11 of Handbook of psychology* (pp. 381–406). Hoboken, NJ: John Wiley & Sons.

Goldstein, N. E., Condie, L. O., Kalbeitzer, R., Osman, D., & Geier, J. (2003). Juvenile offenders' *Miranda* rights comprehension and self-reported likelihood of offering false confessions. *Assessment, 10,* 359–369.

Goldstein, N. E., Condie, L., & Kalbeitzer, R. (2005). Assessing juvenile's competency to waive *Miranda* rights. In T. Grisso, G. Vincent, & D. Seagrave (Eds.), *Handbook for mental health screening and assessment in juvenile justice.* New York: Guilford Publications.

Greenberg, S. A., & Shuman, D. W. (1997). Irreconcilable conflict between therapeutic and forensic roles. *Professional Psychology: Research and Practice, 28,* 50–57.

Greenfield, D. P., Dougherty, E. J., Jackson, R. M., Podboy, J. W., & Zimmerman, M. L. (2001). Retrospective evaluation of *Miranda* reading levels and waiver competency. *American Journal of Forensic Psychology, 19*(2), 75–86.

Grisso, T. (1981). *Juveniles' Waiver of Rights: Legal and Psychological Competence* (Vol. 3). New York: Plenum Publishing Corp.

Grisso, T. (1986). *Evaluating competencies: Forensic assessments and instruments.* New York: Plenum Press.

Grisso, T. (1998). *Forensic evaluation of juveniles.* Sarasota, FL: Professional Resource Press.

Grisso, T. (1998). Instruments for Assessing Understanding and Appreciation of *Miranda* Rights. Sarasota, FL: Professional Resource Press.

Grisso, T. (2003). *Evaluating competencies: Forensic assessments and instruments.* New York: Plenum Press.

Grisso, T. (2004). Reply to "A critical review of competency-to-confess measures." *Law and Human Behavior, 28,* 719–724.

Grisso, T. (Ed.) (2003). *Evaluating competencies: Forensic assessments and instruments* (2nd ed.). New York: Kluwer/Plenum Press.

Grisso, T., & Pomicter, C. (1977). Interrogation of juveniles: An empirical study of procedures, safeguards, and rights waivers. *Law and Human Behavior, 1,* 321–342.

Grisso, T., & Ring, M. (1979). Parents' attitudes toward juveniles' rights in interrogation. *Criminal Justice and Behavior, 6,* 211–226.

Grisso, T., & Schwartz, R. G. (Eds.) (2000). Youth on trial: A developmental Perspective on juvenile justice. Chicago: University of Chicago Press.

Grisso, T., Steinberg, L., Woolard, J., Cauffman, E., Scott, E., Graham, S., Lexcen, F., Reppucci, N. D., & Schwartz, R. (2003). Juveniles' competence to stand trial: A comparison of adolescents' and adults' capacities as trial defendants. *Law & Human Behavior, 27*(4), 333–363.

Gudjonsson, G. H. (1984). A new scale of interrogative suggestibility. *Personality and Individual Differences, 5,* 303–314.

Gudjonsson, G. H. (1987). A parallel form of the Gudjonsson Suggestibility Scale. *British Journal of Clinical Psychology, 26,* 215–221.

Gudjonsson, G. H. (1992). *The psychology of interrogations, confessions and testimony.* New York: John Wiley & Sons.

Gudjonsson, G. H. (1993). Confession evidence, psychological vulnerability and expert testimony. *Journal of Community and Applied Social Psychology, 3,* 117–129.

Gudjonsson, G. H. (1995). 'Fitness for interview' during police detention: A conceptual framework for forensic assessment. *Journal of Forensic Psychiatry, 6,* 185–197.

Gudjonsson, G. H. (1997). *The Gudjonsson Suggestibility Scales Manual.* Hove, U.K.: Psychology Press.

Gudjonsson, G. H., and Clare, I. C. H. (1994). The proposed new police caution (England and Wales): how easy is it to understand? *Expert Evidence, 3,* 109–112.

Gudjonsson, G. H., & Clark, N. K. (1986). Suggestibility in police interrogation: A social psychological model. *Social Behaviour, 1*(2), 83–104.

Gudjonsson, G. H., & Sigurdsson, J. F. (1999). The Gudjonsson Confession Questionnaire-Revised (GCQ-R): Factor structure and its relationship with personality. *Personality and Individual Differences,* *27*(5), 953–968.

Gudjonsson, G. H., & Singh, K. A. (1984). Interrogative suggestibility and delinquent boys: An empirical validation study. *Personality and Individual Differences,* *5*(4), 425–430.

Guy, K. L., & Huckabee, R. G. (1988). Going free on a technicality: Another look at the effect of the *Miranda* decision on the criminal justice process. *Criminal Justice Research Bulletin,* *4*, 1–3.

Harrison, R. J., & Bennett, C. (1995). Racial and ethnic diversity. *State of the Union: America in the 1990s,* *2*, 141–210.

Harrison, Y., & Horne, J. A. (1996). Performance on a complex frontal lobe oriented task with "real-world" significance is impaired following sleep loss. *Journal of Sleep Research,* *5*(1), 87.

Hartley, L., & Shirley, E. (1977). Sleep-loss, noise and decisions. *Ergonomics,* *20*(5), 481–489.

Hays, J. R. (2008). A response to Shealy, Cramer, and Pierlli's "Third Party Presence During Criminal Evaluations": Psychologists' opinions, attitudes, and practices. *Professional Psychology: Research and Practice,* *39*, 570–572.

Heilbrun, K. (1992). The role of psychological testing in forensic assessment. *Law and Human Behavior,* *16*, 257–272.

Heilbrun, K. (2001). *Principles of forensic mental health assessment.* New York: Kluwer/Plenum Publishers.

Heilbrun, K., DeMatteo, D., Marczky, G., & Goldstein, A. M. (2008). Standards of practice and care in forensic mental health assessment: Legal, professional, and principles-based considerations. *Psychology, Public Policy, and Law,* *14*, 1–26.

Heilbrun, K., Grisso, T., & Goldstein, A.M. (2009). *Foundations of forensic mental health assessment.* New York: Oxford University Press.

Heilbrun, K., Marczyk, G. R., & DeMatteo, D. (2002). *Forensic mental health assessment: A casebook.* New York: Oxford University Press.

Heilbrun, K., Warren, J., & Picarello, K. (2003). Third party information in forensic assessment. In A. M. Goldstein (Ed.), *Forensic psychology: Vol. 11 of Handbook of psychology,* (pp. 69–86). Hoboken, NJ: John Wiley & Sons.

Heinrichs, R. W., & Zakzanis, K. K. (1998). Neurocognitive deficit in schizophrenia: A quantitative review of the evidence. *Neuropsychology,* *12*(3), 426–445.

Hess, A. K. (2006). Serving as an expert witness. In I. B. Weiner & A. K. Hess (Eds.), *The handbook of forensic psychology* (3rd ed.), (pp. 652–697). Hoboken, NJ: John Wiley & Sons.

Hockey, G. (1970). Changes in attention allocation in a multicomponent task under loss of sleep. *British Journal of Psychology,* *61*(4), 473–480.

Horn, J. L., & Hofer, S. M. (1992). *Major abilities and development in the adult period.* New York: Cambridge University Press.

Horne, J. A. (1988). Sleep loss and "divergent" thinking ability. *Sleep: Journal of Sleep Research & Sleep Medicine, 11*(6), 528–536.

Hull, J. G., & Young, R. D. (1983). Self-consciousness, self-esteem, and success-failure as determinants of alcohol consumption in male social drinkers. *Journal of Personality and Social Psychology, 44,* 1097–1109.

Inbau, F. E., & Reid, J. E. (1962). *Criminal investigations and confessions.* Baltimore: Williams & Wilkins.

Inbau, F. E., Reid, J. E., & Buckley. J. P. (2003). *Criminal interrogation and confessions* (4th ed.). Baltimore: Williams & Wilkins. *Journal of Forensic Psychiatry, 7,* 297–309.

International Association of Chiefs of Police National Policy Center (January 2004). *Model policy.* Alexandria, VA: IACP

International Association of Chiefs of Police National Policy Center. (April 2004). *Interrogations and confessions: Concepts and issues.* Alexandria, VA: IACP

Juvenile Justice Center (1995). *A Call for Justice: An Assessment of Access to Counsel and Quality of Representation in Delinquency Proceedings.* Washington, DC: American Bar Association, Juvenile Justice Center.

Kalbeitzer, R. (2008). Evaluating legal learning: The effects of time and development on adolescents' understanding of legal rights. *Dissertation Abstracts International, 69,* 1981.

Kalbeitzer, R., Goldstein, N. E. S., Riggs Romaine, C., Mesiarik, C., & Zelle, H. (March 2008). Reliability and validity of the *Miranda* Rights Comprehension Instruments – II. Presented at the annual conference of the *American Psychology–Law Society,* Jacksonville, FL.

Kambam, P., & Thompson, C. (2009). The development of decision-making capacities in children and adolescents: Psychological and neurological perspectives and their implications for juvenile defendants. *Behavioral Sciences and the Law, 27,* 173–190.

Kassin, S. M. (1997). The psychology of confession evidence. *American Psychologist, 52,* 221–233.

Kassin, S. M. (2005). On the psychology of confessions: Does *innocence* put *innocents* at risk? *American Psychologist, 60,* 215–228.

Kassin, S. M., Drizin, S. A., Grisso, T., Gudjonsson, G. H., Leo, R. A., & Redlich, A. D. (2010). Police-induced confessions: Risk factors and recommendations. *Law & Human Behavior, 34,* 3–38.

Kassin, S. M., Leo, R. A., Meissner, C. A., Richman, K. D., Colwell, L. H., Leach, A.-M., et al. (2007). Police interviewing and interrogation: A self-report survey of police practices and beliefs. *Law and Human Behavior, 31*(4), 381–400.

King, C. A., Naylor, M. W., Segal, H. G., Evans, T., & Shain, B.N. (1993). Global self-worth, specific self-perceptions of competence, and depression in adolescents. *Journal of the American Academy of Child and Adolescent Psychiatry, 32* (4), 745–752.

Klaczynski, P. A. (2001). The influence of analytic and heuristic processing on adolescent reasoning and decision making. *Child Development, 72,* 844–861.

Kruh, I., & Grisso, T. (2009). *Evaluation of juveniles' competence to stand trial.* New York: Oxford University Press.

Lally, S. J. (2003). What tests are acceptable for use in forensic evaluations?: A survey of experts. *Professional Psychology - Research & Practice, 34*(5), 491–498.

Law Reform Commission of South Wales. (1998). *The right to silence: Discussion paper 41:.* Online at www.lawlink.nsw.gov.au/lrc.nsf/pages/DP41CHP2.

Leo, R. A. (1996). Inside the interrogation room. *Journal of Criminal Law and Criminology, 86,* 266–276.

Leo, R. A. (2008). *Police interrogation and American justice.* Cambridge, MA: Harvard University Press.

Levin, H. S., Culhane, K. A., Hartmann, J., Evankovich, K., Mattson, A. J., Harward, H., Ringholz, G., Ewing-Cobbs, L., and Fletcher, J. M., 1991. Developmental changes in performance on tests of purported frontal lobe functioning. *Developmental Neuropsychology, 7,* 377–395.

Lezak, M. D. (1983). Neuropsychological assessment (2nd ed.). New York: Oxford University Press.

Lipsitt, P. D. (2007). Ethics and forensic psychological practice. In A. M. Goldstein (Ed.), *Forensic psychology: Emerging topics and expanding roles* (pp. 171–189). Hoboken, NJ: John Wiley & Sons.

Lubet, S. (1998). *Expert testimony: A guide for expert witnesses and lawyers who examine them.* Notre Dame, IN: National Institute for Trial Advocacy.

MacLeod, A.K., Rose, G.S., & Williams, J.M.G. (1993). Components of hopelessness about the future in parasuicide. *Cognitive Therapy and Research, 17*(5), 441–455.

Madden, G. J., Bickel, W. K., & Jacobs, E. A. (1999). Discounting of delayed rewards in opioid-dependent outpatients: Exponential or hyperbolic discounting functions? *Experimental & Clinical Psychopharmacology, 7*(3), 284–293.

McCarthy, M. E., & Waters, W. F. (1997). Decreased attentional responsivity during sleep deprivation: Orienting response latency, amplitude, and habituation. *Sleep: Journal of Sleep Research & Sleep Medicine, 20*(2), 115–123.

McCormick, C. T. (1972). *Handbook of the law of evidence* (2nd ed.). St. Paul, MN: West.

McKay, K. E., Halperin, J. M., Schwartz, S. T., & Sharma, V. (1994). Developmental analysis of three aspects of information processing: Sustained attention, selective attention, and response organization. *Developmental Neuropsychology,10*(2), 121–132.

Melton, G. B. (2008). Beyond balancing: Toward an integrated approach to children's rights. *Journal of Social Issues, 64*(4), 903–920.

Melton, G. B., Petrila, J., Poythress, N. G., & Slobogin, C. (2007). *Psychological evaluations for the courts: A handbook for mental health professionals and lawyers* (3rd ed.). New York: The Guilford Press.

Messenheimer, S., Riggs Romaine, C.L., Wolbransky, M., Zelle, H., Serico, J. M., Wrazien, L., & Goldstein, N.E.S., (2009). Readability and comprehension: A comparison of the two versions of the *Miranda* rights assessment instruments. Presented at the annual conference of the *American Psychology– Law Society*, San Antonio, TX.

Mineka, S., Rafaeli, E., Yovel, I. (2003) Cognitive biases in emotional disorders: Information processing and social-cognitive perspectives. In: R. J. Davidson, K. R. Scherer, & H. H. Goldsmith (Eds), *Handbook of affective sciences* (pp. 976–1009). Oxford: Oxford University Press.

Moston, S., Stephenson, G. M., & Williamson, T. M. (1992). The effects of case characteristics on suspect behaviour during police questioning. *British Journal of Criminology, 32*, 23–40.

Nardulli, P. F. (1983). The societal costs of the exclusionary rule: An empirical assessment. *American Bar Foundation Research Journal, 8*, 585–609.

Nardulli, P. F. (1987). The societal costs of the exclusionary rule revisited. *University of Illinois Law Review, 2*, 223–239.

Norton, R. (1970). The effects of acute sleep deprivation on selective attention. *British Journal of Psychology, 61*, 157–161.

Oberlander, L. B. (1998). *Miranda* comprehension and professional competence. *Expert Opinion, 2*, 11–12.

Oberlander, L. B., & Goldstein, N. E. (2001). A review and update in the practice of evaluating *Miranda* comprehension. *Behavioral Sciences and the Law, 19*, 453–471.

Oberlander, L. B., Goldstein, N. E., & Goldstein, A.M. (2003). Competence to confess. In A. M. Goldstein, (Ed.), *Forensic psychology*, Vol. 11 of the *Handbook of Psychology*, pp. 335–357. Hoboken, NJ: John Wiley & Sons.

O'Connell, M. J., Garmoe, W., & Goldstein, N. E. (2005). *Miranda* comprehension in adults with mental retardation and the effects of feedback style on suggestibility. *Law and Human Behavior, 29*(3), 359–369.

Olley, M. C. (1998). The utility of the test of charter comprehension for ensuring the protection of accuseds' rights at the time of arrest. Unpublished doctoral dissertation, Simon Fraser University, Burnaby, British Columbia, Canada.

Olley, M. C., Ogloff, J. R., & Jager, L. (1993). Do people understand their rights when arrested? The test of charter comprehension. *Rehabilitation Review, 4*, 1–2.

Olubadewo, Oluseyi (2009). The relationship between mental health symptoms and comprehension of *Miranda* rights in male juvenile offenders. *Dissertation Abstracts International, 69*, 5788.

Otto, R. K., Slobogin, C., & Greenberg, S. A. (2007). Legal and ethical issues in accessing and utilizing third-party information. In A. M. Goldstein (Ed.), *Forensic psychology: Emerging topics and expanding roles* (pp. 190–208). Hoboken, NJ: John Wiley & Sons.

Otto, R. K., & Goldstein, A. M. (2005). Juveniles' competence to confess and competence to participate in the juvenile justice process. In K. Heilbrun, N. E. S.Goldstein, & R. E. Redding (Eds.), *Juvenile delinquency: Prevention, assessment, and intervention* (pp. 179–208). New York: Oxford University Press.

Packer, I. K. (2009). *Evaluation of criminal responsibility.* NY: Oxford University Press.

Pearse, J. (1995). Police interviewing: The identification of vulnerabilities. *Journal of Community and Applied Social Psychology, 5,* 147–159.

Pearse, J., & Gudjonsson, G. (1997). Police interviewing and legal representation: A field study. *Journal of Forensic Psychiatry & Psychology, 8*(1), 200–208.

Pearse, J., Gudjonsson, G. H., Clare, I. C. H., & Rutter, S. (1998). Police interviewing and psychological vulnerabilities: Predicting the likelihood of a confession. *Journal of Community and Applied Social Psychology, 8,* 1–21.

Pelham, B. W., & Neter, E. (1995). The effect of motivation of judgment depends on the difficulty of the judgment. *Journal of Personality & Social Psychology, 68*(4), 581–594.

Peterson-Badali, M., Abramovitch, R., Koegl, C. J., & Ruck, M. D. (1999). Young people's experience of the Canadian youth justice system: Interacting with police and legal counsel. *Behavioral Sciences & the Law, 17*(4), 455–465.

Pogrebin, M. R. & Poole, E. D. (1987). Deinstitutionalization and increased arrest rates among the mentally disordered. *Journal of Psychiatry and Law, 15,* 117–127.

Randazzo, A. C., Muehlbach, M. J., Schweitzer, P. K., & Walsh, J. K. (1998). Cognitive function following acute sleep restriction in children ages 10-14. *Sleep: Journal of Sleep Research & Sleep Medicine, 21*(8), 861–868.

Redding, R. E. (2006). The brain-disordered defendant: Neuroscience and legal insanity in the twenty-first century. *American University Law Review, 56,* 51–127.

Redding, R. E., Floyd, M. Y., & Hawk, G. L. (2001). What judges and lawyers think about the testimony of mental health experts: A survey of the courts and bar. *Behavioral Sciences and the Law, 19,* 583–594.

Richardson, G., Gudjonsson, G. H., & Kelly, T. P. (1995). Interrogative suggestibility in an adolescent forensic population. *Journal of Adolescence 18,* 211–216.

Riggs Romaine, C. L., Zelle, H., Wolbransky, M., Zelechoski, A. D., & Goldstein, N. E. S. (2008). Juveniles' *Miranda* rights comprehension: Comparing understanding in two states. Poster presented at the annual convention of the *American Psychological Association,* Boston, MA.

Robertson, G., Pearson, R., & Gibb, R. (1996). Police interviewing and the use of appropriate adults. *Journal of Forensic Psychiatry, 7,* 297–309.

Rogers, R. (2008a). An introduction to response styles. In R. Rogers (Ed.), *Clinical assessment of malingering and deception* (3rd ed.), (pp. 3–13). NY: Guilford Press.

Rogers, R. (Ed.). (2008b). *Clinical assessment of malingering and deception* (3rd ed.). NY: Guilford Press.

Rogers, R. (2008c). Structured interviews and dissimulation. In R. Rogers (Ed.), *Clinical assessment of malingering and deception* (3rd ed.), (pp. 301–322). NY: Guilford Press.

Rogers, R., Correa, A. A., Hazelwood, L. L., Shuman, D. W., Hoersting, R. C., & Blackwood, H. L. (2009). Spanish translations of *Miranda* warnings and the totality of the circumstances. *Law and Human Behavior, 33,* 61–69.

Rogers, R., & Ewing, C. P. (1989). Ultimate opinion proscriptions: A cosmetic fix and a plea for empiricism. *Law and Human Behavior, 13,* 357–374.

Rogers, R., Harrison, K. S., Hazelwood, L. L., & Sewell, K. W. (2007). Knowing and intelligent: A study of *Miranda* warnings in mentally disordered defendants. *Law and Human Behavior, 31,* 401–418.

Rogers, R., Harrison, K. S., Shuman, D. W., Sewell, K. W., & Hazelwood, L. L. (2007). An analysis of *Miranda* warnings and waivers: Comprehension and coverage. *Law and Human Behavior, 31,* 177–192.

Rogers, R., Hazelwood, L. L., Sewell, K. W., Blackwood, H. L., Rogstad, J. E., & Harrison, K. S. (2009). Development and initial validation of the Miranda Vocabulary Scale. *Law and Human Behavior, 33,* 381–392.

Rogers, R., Hazelwood, L.L., Sewell, K.W., Harrison, K.S., Shuman, D.W. (2008). The language of *Miranda* warnings in American jurisdictions: A replication and vocabulary analysis. *Law and Human Behavior, 32,* 124–136.

Rogers, R., Hazelwood, L. L., Sewell, K. W., Shuman, D. W., & Blackwood, H. L. (2008). The comprehensibility and content of juvenile *Miranda* warnings. *Psychology, Public Policy, and Law, 14,* 63–87.

Rogers, R., Jordan, M. J., & Harrison, K. S. (2004). A critical review of published competency-to-confess measures. *Law and Human Behavior, 28,* 707–718.

Rogers, R., Salekin, R. T., Sewell, K. W., Goldstein, A. M., & Leonard, K. (1998). A comparison of forensic and nonforensic malingerers: A prototypical analysis of explanatory models. *Law and Human Behavior, 22,* 353–367.

Rogers, R., Sewell, K. W., & Goldstein, A. M. (1994). Explanatory models of malingering: A prototypical analysis. *Law and Human Behavior, 18,* 543–552.

Rogers, R., & Shuman, D. (2005). *Fundamentals of forensic practice: Mental health and criminal law.* New York: Springer.

Rosner, R. (Ed.). (2003). *Principles and practice of forensic psychiatry* (2nd ed.). NY: Oxford University Press.

Ruback, R. B., & Vardaman, P. J. (1997). Decision making in delinquency cases: The role of race and juveniles' admission/denial of the Crime. *Law & Human Behavior, 21*(1), 47–69.

Ryan, C. M. (1990). "Age-related improvement in short-term memory efficiency during adolescence." *Developmental Neuropsychology 6*(3), 193–205.

Ryba, N. L., Brodsky, S. L., & Shlosberg, A. (2007). Evaluations of capacity to waive *Miranda* rights: A survey of practitioners' use of the Grisso instruments. *Assessment, 14*(3), 300–309.

Saks, M. J. (1990). Expert witnesses, nonexpert witnesses, and nonwitness experts. *Law and Human Behavior, 14,* 291–313.

Salekin, R. T., Rogers, R., & Ustad, K. L. (2001). Juvenile waiver to adult criminal courts: Prototypes for dangerousness, sophistication-maturity, and amenability to treatment. *Psychology, Public Policy, and Law, 7*(2), 381–408.

Salekin, R. T., Yff, R. M. A., Neumann, C. S., Leistico, A. R., & Zalot, A. A. (2002). Juvenile transfer to adult courts: A look at the prototypes for dangerousness, sophistication-maturity, and amenability to treatment through a legal lens. *Psychology, Public Policy, and Law, 8*(4), 373–410.

Schellenberg, E., Wasylenki, D., Webster, C. D., & Goering, P. (1992) A review of arrests among psychiatric patients. *International Journal of Law and Psychiatry, 15*(3), 251–264.

Scott, E. S., Reppucci, D., & Woolard, J. L. (1995). Evaluating adolescent decision making in legal contexts. *Law and Human Behavior, 19*(3), 221–244.

Shapiro, D. L. (1991). *Forensic psychological assessment: An integrative approach.* Needham Heights, MA: Allyn and Bacon.

Shaw, J. A., & Budd, E. C. (1982). Determinants of acquiescence and naysaying of mentally retarded persons. *American Journal of Mental Deficiency, 87*(1), 108–110.

Shealy, C., Cramer, R. J., & Pirielli, G. (2008). Third party presence during criminal forensic evaluations: Psychologists' opinions, attitudes, and practices. *Professional Psychology: Research and Practice, 39,* 561–569.

Shepherd, E. W., Mortimer, A. K., & Mobasheri, R. (1995). The police caution: Comprehension and perceptions in the general population. *Expert Evidence, 4,* 60–67.

Shuy, R. W. (1998). *The language of confession, interrogation, and deception.* Thousand Oaks, CA: Sage Press.

Simon, R. I., & Gold, L. H. (2004). *American Psychiatric Publishing textbook of forensic psychiatry.* Washington, D.C.: American Psychiatry Publishing.

Slobogin, C. (1989). The "ultimate issue" issue. *Behavioral Sciences and the Law, 7,* 259–266.

Sowell, E. R., Thompson, P. M., Holmes, C. J., Jernigan, T. L., & Toga, A. W. (1999). In vivo evidence for post-adolescent brain maturation in frontal and striatal regions. *Nature Neuroscience, 2,* 859–861.

Steinberg, L. (2008). A social neuroscience perspective on adolescent risk-taking. *Developmental Review, 28*(1), 78–106.

Steinberg, L. & Monahan, K. (2007). Age differences in resistance to peer influence. *Developmental Psychology, 43,* 1531–1543.

Steinberg, L., & Cauffman, E. (1996). Maturity of judgment in adolescence: Psychosocial factors in adolescent decision making. *Law & Human Behavior, 20*(3), 249–272.

Sweet, J. J., Condit, D. C., & Nelson, N. W. (2008). Feigned amnesia and memory loss. In R. Rogers (Ed.), *Clinical assessment of malingering and deception* (3rd ed.) (pp. 218–236). NY: Guilford Press.

Teplin, L. A. (1983). The criminalization of the mentally ill: Speculation in search of data. *Psychological Bulletin, 94*(1), 54–67.

Teplin, LA. (2000). *Keeping the Peace: Police Discretion and Mentally Ill Persons.* NIJ Journal.Washington, DC: National Institute of Justice.

Toren, P., Sadeh, M., Wolmer, L., Eldare, S., Koren, S., Weizman, R., & Laor, N. (2000). Neurocognitive correlates of anxiety disorders in children: A preliminary report. *Journal of Anxiety Disorders, 14*(3), 239–247.

Viljoen, J. L., & Roesch, R. (2005). Competence to waive interrogation rights and adjudicative competence in adolescent defendants: Cognitive development, attorney contact, and psychological symptoms. *Law & Human Behavior, 26*(5), 481–506.

Viljoen, J. L., Klaver, J., & Roesch, R. (2005). Legal decisions of preadolescent and adolescent defendants: Predictors of confessions, pleas, communication with attorneys, and appeals. *Law & Human Behavior, 29*(3), 253–277.

Viljoen, J. L., Roesch, R., & Zapf, P. A. (2002). An examination of the relationship between competency to stand trial, competency to waive interrogation rights, and psychopathology. *Law & Human Behavior, 26*(5), 481–506.

Weissman, H., & DeBow, D. (2003). Ethical principles and professional competencies. In A. M. Goldstein (Ed.), *Forensic psychology:* Vol. 11 of *Handbook of psychology* (pp. 33–54). Hoboken, NJ: John Wiley & Sons.

White, W. S. (2001). *Miranda's waning protections: Police interrogation practices after Dickerson.* Ann Arbor, MI: University of Michigan Press.

Williams, H. L., Lubin, A., & Goodnow, J. J. (1959). Impaired performance with acute sleep loss. *Psychological Monographs: General and Applied, 73,* 1–26.

Wimmer, F., Hoffmann, R. F., Bonato, R. A., & Moffitt, A. R. (1992). The effects of sleep deprivation on divergent thinking and attention processes. *Journal of Sleep Research, 1,* 223–230.

Winick, B. J. (1996). *Incompetency to proceed in the criminal process: Past, present, and future.* Belmont, CA: Thomson Brooks/Cole Publishing Co.

Witt, P. H., & Conroy, M. A. (2009). *Evaluation of sexually violent predators.* New York: Oxford University Press.

Wood, J., & Crawford, A. (1989). *The right to remain silent.* London: Civil Liberties Trust.

Wrightman, L. S., & Kassin, S. M. (1993). *Confessions in the courtroom.* Newbury Park, CA: Sage Press.

Zapf, P., & Roesch, R. (2009). *Evaluation of competence to stand trial.* New York: Oxford University Press.

Zelle, H., Goldstein, N. E. S., Riggs Romaine, C., Serico, J., & Taormina, S. (2008). Factor structure of the *Miranda* Rights Comprehension Instruments – II. Presented at the annual conference of the *American Psychology–Law Society,* Jacksonville, FL.

Zelle, H., Riggs Romaine, C. L., Serico, J. M., Wolbransky, M., Osman, D. A., Taormina, S., Wrazien, L., & Goldstein, N. E. S. (August 2008). Adolescents' *Miranda* rights comprehension: The impact of verbal expressive abilities. Presented at the annual conference of the *American Psychological Association,* Boston, MA.

Ziskin, J. (1995). *Coping with psychiatric and psychological testimony* (5th ed., Vols. 1–3). Beverly Hills, CA: Law and Psychology Press.

Ziskin, J. (2000). *2000 Supplement to coping with psychiatric and psychological testimony* (5th ed.). Los Angles: Law and Psychology Press.

Tests and Specialized Tools

CMR: Comprehension of Miranda Rights (Grisso, 1998)

CMR-R: Comprehension of Miranda Rights–Recognition (Grisso, 1998

CMV: Comprehension of Miranda Vocabulary (Grisso, 1998)

FRI: Function of Rights in Interrogation (Grisso, 1998)

MRCI-II: Miranda Rights Comprehension Instruments – II (Goldstein, Zelle, & Grisso, in preparation)

WAIS-III: Wechsler Adult Intelligence Scale (Wechsler, 1997)

References

Goldstein, N. E. S., Zelle, H., & Grisso, T. (in preparation). *Miranda Rights Comprehension Instruments – II*. Sarasota, FL: Professional Resource Press.

Grisso, T. (1998). *Instruments for assessing understanding and appreciation of Miranda rights*. Sarasota, FL: Professional Resource Press.

Wechsler, D. (1997). *WAIS-III administration and scoring manual*. San Antonio, TX: Psychological Corporation.

Cases and Statutes

Brown v. Mississippi, 297 U.S. 278 (1936)
Brown v. Walker, 161 U. S. 591 (1896)
California v. Prysock, 453 U.S. 355 (1981)
Colorado v. Connelly, 479 U.S. 157 (1986)
Commonwealth v. Day, 387 Mass. 915, 920, 921; 444 N.E.2d
384 (1983)
Commonwealth v. Jackson, 432 Mass. 82, 85; 731 N.E. 2d 1066
(2000)
Commonwealth v. Mandile, 497 Mass. 410 (1986)
Commonwealth v. Meehan, 377 Mass. 522 (1979)
Commonwealth v. Soares, 745 N.E. 2d 362, Mass. App. Ct.
(2000)
Coyote v. United States, 380 F. 2d. 305 (1967)
Crane v. Kentucky, 476 U.S. 683 (1986)
Culombe v. Connecticut, 367 U.S. 568 (1961)
Daubert v. Merrell Dow Pharmaceutical, 509 U.S. 579 (1993)
Dickerson v. United States, 530 U.S. 428 (2000)
Escobedo v. Illinois, 378 U.S. 478 (1964)
Estelle v. Smith, 451 U.S. 454, 101 S. Ct. 1866 (1981)
Fare v. Michael C., 442 U.S. 707 (1979)
Fellers v. United States, 540 U.S. 519 (2004)
Frazier v. Cupp. 394 U.S. 731 (1969)
Frye v. United States, 293 F. 1013 (1923)
Gallegos v. Colorado, 370 U.S. 49 (1962)
Garner v. Mitchell, 2007 U. S. App. Lexis 21705; 2007 Fed. App.
0370P (6th Cir.), (2007)
Hahn v. Union Pacific Railroad, IL Appellate Court, 5th District,
No. 5-03-0466, decision filed 09-24-04 (Unpublished)
Haley v. Ohio, 332 U.S. 596 (1948)
Hayes v. Washington, 373 U.S. 503 (1963)
Hopt v. Territory of Utah, 104 U.S. 631 (1884)
In re Gault, 387 U.S. 1 (1967)
In re Patrick W., 84 Cal.App.3d 529 (1978)
Jackson v. Denno, 378 US 368 (1964)

Jenkins v. United States, 309 F.2d 852, 854 (1962)
Johnson v. Zerbst, 304 U.S. 458 (1938)
Kent v. United States, 383 U.S. 541 (1966)
Lego v. Twomey, 404 US 477 (1972)
Miranda v. Arizona, 384 U.S. 436 (1966)
Misskelley v. State, 323 Ark. 449, 915 S.W. 2d 702 (1996)
Missouri v. Siebert, 542 U.S. 600 (2004)
Moran v. Burbine, 475 US 412 (1986)
Morris v. State, 1988 Okla. Crim. 298, 766, P.2d 1388 (1988)
Oregon v. Elstad, 470 US 298 (1985)
People v. Al-Yousif, 49 P.3d 1165 (2002)
People v. Baker, 92 Ill. 2d 85, 90 (1973)
People v. Bennett, 876 N.E. 2d 256 (2007)
People v. Bernasco, 138 Ill.2d 349 (1990)
People v. Cronin, 60 NY2d 430, 433 (1983)
People v. Daoud, 462 Mich. 621, 643; 614 N.W.2d 152 (2000)
People v. Hernandez, 46 A.D.3d 574, 846 N.W.S.2d 371 (2007)
People v. Higgins, 278 N.E.2d 68 (1993)
People v. Huntley, 15 NY2d 72 (1965)
People v. Kogut, 10 Misc. 3d 305; 806 NY2d 366 (2005)
People v. Lara, 432 P.2d 202 (1967)
People v. Marx, 305 AD2d. 726 (2003)
People v. Trujillo, 938 P.2d 117 (1993)
People v. Williams, 62 NY2d. 285 (1984)
Schneckloth v. Busamonte, 412 U.S. 218 (1973)
Spano v. New York, 360 U.S. 315 (1958)
State v. Anderson, 404 N.W.2d 856, 858 (1987)
State v. Coombs, 704 A.2d 387, 392 (1998)
State v. Kelly, 603 S.W.2d 726, 728 (1980)
State v. Mikulewicz, 462 A.2d 497, 501 (1983)
State v. Romero, (Case No. A111035, OR. Ct. App.) (2003)
United States ex rel. Simon v. Maroney, 228 F. Supp. 800 (1964)
United States v. Crocker, 510 F.2d 1129 (1975)
United States v. Inman, 352 F.2d 954 (1965)
United States v. Raposo, 1998 WL 879723 (1998)
United States v. Wade, 388 U.S. 218 (1967)
West v. United States, 399 F.2d 467 (1968) (1968)

Key Terms

Daubert standard: states that evidence based on innovative or unusual scientific knowledge may be admitted only after it has been established that the evidence is reliable and scientifically valid. Defined a gatekeeping function for judges in which they consider testing, peer review, error rates, and underlying science to determine admissibility of evidence.

exculpatory statement: a statement or other evidence that tends to justify, excuse, or clear a defendant from an alleged fault or guilt.

Gudjonsson Suggestibility Scales (GSS): developed by Gisli H. Gudjonsson, the GSS is a test that tries to measure how susceptible a person is to coercive interrogation. It relies on two different aspects of interrogative suggestibility: *yielding* to leading questions; and *shifting* responses when interrogative pressure is applied.

Frye standard: provides that expert opinion based on a scientific technique is admissible only where the technique is generally accepted as reliable in the relevant scientific community.

inculpatory statement: a confession or statement of guilt.

informed consent: an individual's consent for another person to engage in intervention that would otherwise constitute an invasion of the individual's privacy, after the individual has been fully informed of the nature and consequences of the proposed action, is competent to consent, and consents voluntarily. Informed consent is not necessary on court-ordered or statutorily mandated evaluations in criminal or delinquency cases, or when authorized by legal counsel for the individual.

Instruments for Assessing Understanding and Appreciation of *Miranda* Rights: Four assessment measures developed by Dr. Thomas Grisso to help mental health professionals assess the capacity of juvenile and adult defendants to appreciate and understand the significance of their *Miranda* rights. The four instruments are: Comprehension of Miranda Rights (CMR); Comprehension of Miranda Rights–Recognition (CMR-R);

Comprehension of Miranda Vocabulary (CMV); and Function of Rights in Interrogation (FRI).

Miranda rights: protects an individual's Fifth Amendment right against self-incrimination (the right to remain silent) and Sixth Amendment right to have an attorney present before and during police questioning (the right to an attorney).

suppression hearing: a hearing on a criminal defendant's motion to prohibit the prosecutor's use of evidence alleged to have been obtained in violation of the defendant's rights.

totality of circumstances test: a test used to determine whether certain constitutional rights of a defendant have been violated. The test looks to all the circumstances attending the alleged violation, rather than to any particular factors.

trier of fact: refers to the judge or the jury charged with reaching a legal determination in a case.

Index

About the Authors

Alan M. Goldstein, Ph.D., is Professor of Psychology on the graduate faculty of John Jay College of Criminal Justice and on the doctoral faculty of the Clinical Psychology Ph.D. Program at the Graduate Center–City University of New York. He chaired the Continuing Education Program of the American Academy of Forensic Psychology for 20 years. He is President of the American Board of Forensic Psychology, served as Chair of the Ethics Committee of the American Board of Professional Psychology, and was Chair of APA's Continuing Professional Education Committee. Dr. Goldstein is a member of the Board of Trustees of the America Board of Professional Psychology. He is editor of *Forensic Psychology* (2003) and *Forensic Psychology: Emerging Topics and Expanding Roles* (2007), both published by John Wiley and Sons. With Tom Grisso and Kirk Heilbrun, he is the series editor for Best Practices in Forensic Mental Health Assessment, published by Oxford University Press. In addition to this book in that series, he is coauthor of *Foundations of Forensic Mental Health Assessment*. Dr. Goldstein is on the editorial boards of *Behavioral Sciences and the Law* and *Criminal Justice and Behavior*. Dr. Goldstein is Board Certified in Forensic Psychology by the American Board of Professional Psychology. He is in independent practice, conducting forensic assessments on a range of criminal and civil psycholegal issues. He is the recipient of the 1997 Distinguished Contribution Award to the Field of Forensic Psychology from the American Academy of Forensic Psychology. Dr. Goldstein was named the 2000 Continuing Education Distinguished Speaker by the American Psychological Association. He received the Beth Clark Distinguished Service Award to Forensic Psychology in 2006, given by the American Board of Forensic Psychology and in 2007, he received the Distinguished Contribution Award to the American Board of Professional Psychology.

Naomi E. S. Goldstein, Ph.D., is Associate Professor of Psychology at Drexel University and a member of the core faculty of the J.D.-Ph.D. Program in Law and Psychology at Drexel University. She is the former co-Director of the J.D.-Ph.D. Program in Law and Psychology at Villanova School of Law and Drexel University. Dr. Goldstein specializes in juvenile forensic psychology, and she conducts research on adolescents' comprehension of *Miranda* rights and their likelihood of offering true and false confessions to police. Along with Tom Grisso and Heather Zelle, Dr. Goldstein created the *Miranda Rights Comprehension Instruments – II*, the revised version of the *Instruments for Assessing Understanding and Appreciation of Miranda Rights*. Dr. Goldstein's research team has also created the *Miranda Rights Educational Curriculum* and is evaluating its effectiveness in teaching youth about legal rights and legal decision-making. Dr. Goldstein also specializes in the development and evaluation of intervention programs for adolescent female offenders. With a K23 award from the National Institute of Mental Health, she developed the Juvenile Justice Anger Management (JJAM) Treatment for Girls and is evaluating its efficacy in reducing anger, aggressive behaviors, and recidivism rates among female juvenile offenders. Dr. Goldstein's research has been funded by grants and contracts from the National Institute of Mental Health, American Psychology–Law Society, American Academy of Forensic Psychology, Institute for Women's Health at Drexel University, and Philadelphia Department of Human Services. She is on the editorial boards of *Law and Human Behavior*; *Psychology, Public Policy, and the Law*; and *Behavioral Sciences and the Law*. She formerly served on the editorial board of *Criminal Justice and Behavior*, and she served as an Associate Editor of the *Journal of Forensic Psychology Practice*. Along with Kirk Heilbrun and Richard Redding, she is coauthor of the book *Juvenile Delinquency*. Dr. Goldstein holds a B.A in Psychology from Wesleyan University and completed her Ph.D. in Clinical Psychology at the University of Massachusetts, Amherst. Dr. Goldstein completed a clinical internship at the University of Massachusetts Medical Center.